HAIRTALK

Long before the people of the modern world began adding synthetic hair, human hair, or yaki hair to their natural hair, in Africa we had our own type of hair extensions. Being people who were close to the earth, we used the earth to extend and even to color our hair. We used the palms from the trees, shredding them into fine yellow threads. And deep in the jungle there stands a tree, the Cotar tree, on which grows a particular fruit. We used the juice of this fruit to dye the palm strands black. And that was the beginning of hair extensions and colored hair as we know them today.

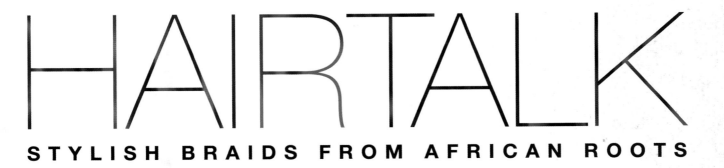

HAIRTALK

STYLISH BRAIDS FROM AFRICAN ROOTS

DUYAN JAMES

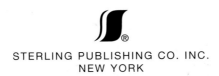

STERLING PUBLISHING CO. INC.
NEW YORK

Library of Congress Cataloging-in-Publication Data Available

10 9 8 7 6 5 4 3 2 1

Published by Sterling Publishing Co., Inc.
387 Park Avenue South, New York, NY 10016

© 2007 by Duyan James

Distributed in Canada by Sterling Publishing
c/o Canadian Manda Group, 165 Dufferin Street
Toronto, Ontario, Canada M6K 3H6

Distributed in the United Kingdom by GMC Distribution Services
Castle Place, 166 High Street, Lewes, East Sussex, England BN7 1XU

Distributed in Australia by Capricorn Link (Australia) Pty. Ltd.
P.O. Box 704, Windsor, NSW 2756, Australia

Printed in China
All rights reserved

Sterling ISBN-13: 978-1-4027-4235-4
        ISBN-10: 1-4027-4235-5

For information about custom editions, special sales, premium and
corporate purchases, please contact Sterling Special Sales
Department at 800-805-5489 or specialsales@sterlingpub.com.

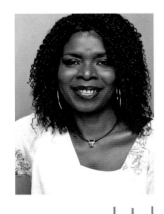

Black women throughout the ages have been connected to one another by many things, the most obvious and prominent of which is hair. We've twisted; we've turned; we've braided. We've gelled it down; we've cornrowed it back. We've done everything imaginable to our hair. Our story of hair goes back before civilization, before the modern world recognized its beauty and its brilliance.

In America, we often view hair only in terms of fashion and style, but in some West African countries, such as Liberia, where I'm from, some hairstyles have deeper meanings. These hairstyles are used for tribal celebration, to ward off the bad spirits, and to mark a coming of age, among many other ritualistic meanings. And, of course, there are styles that are just for fashion.

Most people who are interested in getting their hair done know only that they want to get their hair braided. This book is designed to give the consumer ideas about the types of hairstyles available, details about those styles, and some background information as well. It also provides hair-care advice and tips for creating your own hairstyles.

My braidery, in Washington, D.C., is where these brilliant hairstyles and many wonderful relationships were born. To me, a braidery is more than just a place where you get your hair done. It is also a spiritual and somewhat ritualistic meeting place, a cross-cultural intersection, where minds meet, discuss, argue, and share. My salon hosts braiders from many different jurisdictions in West Africa and abroad. They are from many different tribes, speak many different languages, and have very different backgrounds. Our American customers are just as diverse. Despite our differences, we are always in complete fellowship, as we learn and share our experiences with one another.

There is nothing like the looks on my customers' faces when they leave the salon—transformed. It has been said that when your hair looks good, you feel good on the inside. I know this to be true—I've witnessed it. A little hair magic can take you a long way.

CONTENTS

Hairstyles Created with Natural Hair

Pixies

Specialty Hairstyles

Children's Hairstyles

ACKNOWLEDGMENTS

Special thanks and recognition to:

Braiders
Kine
Mime
Timathy
Mado
Bobo
Bijuo
Cou Cou
Anna
Anna D.
Ester
Badjegue
Aicha
Hadja
Madeleine
Djouweratou

Hair and Makeup
Bathilde Diouf

Photography
Ramon Gaskin
James Hicks
Tony Hawkins

Photography Design
New Millennium Graphics Design and Marketing

Writing
Raquis Da'Juan Petree

HAIRTALK

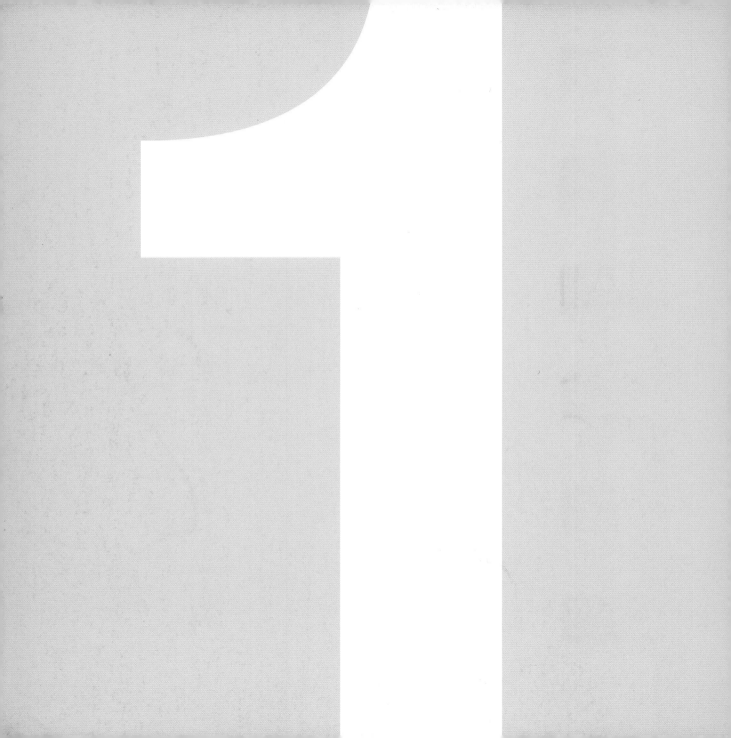

HAIR PREPARATION AND BRAIDING TECHNIQUES

Unless otherwise specified, all descriptions here assume that you are adding yarn or synthetic, pony, or human hair to natural hair.

About the Hair

Women today have more options than ever when it comes to hair extensions. Synthetic hair is the most commonly used. It is inexpensive and comes in a variety of solid colors as well as in two-tone styles. Pony hair is also synthetic hair, but it looks more like human hair and is therefore more expensive than regular synthetic hair. Both regular synthetic hair and pony hair are available at beauty supply stores. Human hair, also available at beauty supply stores, is the most expensive option and is used infrequently. Finally, yarn is used in some styles and is the least expensive of all.

Hair Preparation

Hair should be washed, then dried, before you begin any of the braiding techniques. You will need a comb for parting the hair and clips for holding aside the hair that's not being braided. For some styles you will need thread, yarn, or gel. For weaving you'll need a darning needle and thread.

Styling Preparation

Before you begin, you must have a plan or a design for the style. How many braids will you create? What size will they be? In what direction and at what angle will the braids sit? There are so many ways to part and braid hair! Be sure you know what you want the final style to look like before you begin. Use the size chart included here to help you make your design decisions.

Caring for Your Hair

Some people grease their hair heavily, which can cause their pores to clog and their scalps to itch. Your scalp has to breathe, so it's better to use a light natural oil to condition your scalp. Don't overdo it!

The Hairstyles

Hairstyles can take anywhere from two hours for simple braids to eight or more hours for complex styles. Of course, if more than one person is working on a single style, the time required will be reduced.

The recommended length of time to leave braids in depends on the style. Generally, for cornrows, about one month is recommended. Individual braids, Senegalese twists, and kinky twists can be

For all braiding styles that join yarn or synthetic or pony hair to natural hair, the most important step is joining the synthetic hair or yarn to the natural hair by tightly braiding or twisting the two together.

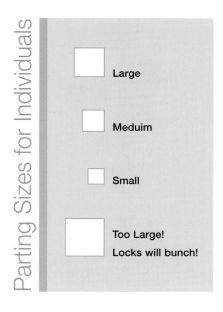

Parting Sizes for Individuals

☐ Large

☐ Meduim

☐ Small

☐ Too Large!
Locks will bunch!

left in for about two months; after that, for these styles, the braids begin to loosen, and everyday wear and tear begins to roughen the look. Refer to the individual styles for information on how long each can be kept in.

The first step for any hairstyle is to plan. When you are happy with your intended style, section the hair as planned, braiding or clipping to the side the hair that's not being worked on right away.

HOW TO CREATE THE STYLES

The author favors and practices all the techniques described here, but methods can vary, and stylists should choose those that are most comfortable for them. Use the descriptions here as a starting point. No chemicals or perms were used to create these styles. Any straightened natural hair was straightened with a flat iron.

When you add human hair extensions to natural hair, you must braid or twist the hair in, as you would with synthetic hair or yarn, and then you must also tie the extension or glue it with nail glue once you have twisted or braided beyond the length of the natural hair. Human hair is softer and more slippery than synthetic hair, and the extension will slip out if it's not glued or tied in place.

Joining Extensions to Natural Hair—Twists

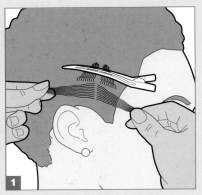

1. To join extensions to natural hair with twists, part the natural hair to create two sections (the amount of extension hair you begin with will depend on the size of the twists or cornrows you want).

2. Divide the lock of hair or yarn that you're adding into two sections and interlock them.

3. Join the pieces in each hand, so you are holding one lock of extension hair in each hand. These will make up the two parts of the twist.

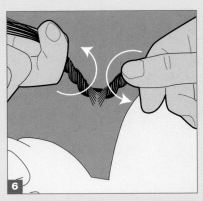

4. Place the interlocking point of the added hair around the two sections of natural hair, next to the scalp.

5. Join one side of the added hair or yarn to one section of the natural hair. Repeat on the other side.

6. Holding one section in each hand, tightly twist about an inch of the hair between your thumb and fingers.

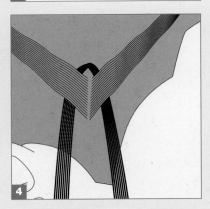

7. Coil the two twisted sections tightly around each other once, carefully moving the hair in your left hand to your right hand, and vice versa. Be sure the twists and coils remain tight.

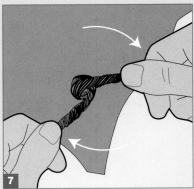

8. Continue this process until you have reached the end of the natural hair; then continue with your intended style. If you are adding human hair extensions, you must tie or glue the extension at the point where you have passed the natural hair, or it will slip out. Nail glue works well. The glue is cut out when the extensions are removed.

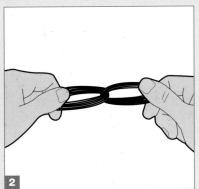

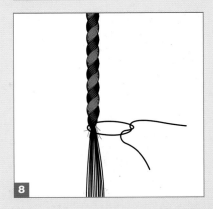

Joining Extensions to Natural Hair—Braids

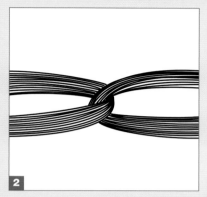

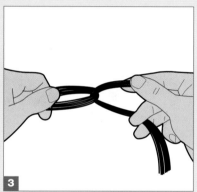

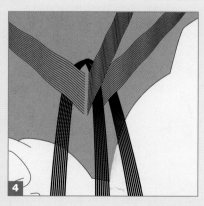

1. To join extensions to natural hair by braiding, begin with three sections of extension hair (the amount of extension hair you begin with will depend on the size of the braids—see size chart on page 5—or cornrows you want).

2. Divide the hair that you're adding into two sections and interlock them.

3. You will be holding two ends of extension hair in each hand. In one hand, keep those two ends separate; in the other hand join the ends together, so you are holding a total of three sections of extension hair—one in one hand and two in the other. These will make up the three parts of the braid.

4. Place the intersection point of the extension hair next to the target sections of natural hair, next to the scalp.

5. Holding the synthetic hair in place with one finger, join one piece of the extension hair to one section of natural hair. Repeat for the other two sections as you braid the extension hair tightly into the natural hair.

6. Press the hair against the scalp with your fingers to be sure the braid remains tight at all times.

7. Continue braiding tightly until you have reached the end of the natural hair; then continue with your intended style. If you are adding human hair extensions, you must tie or glue the extensions once you have braided beyond the natural hair, or they will slip out. Nail glue works well. The glue is cut out when the extensions are removed.

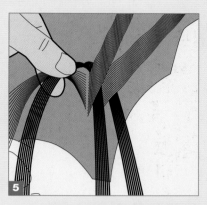

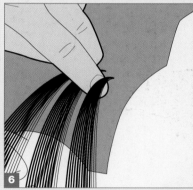

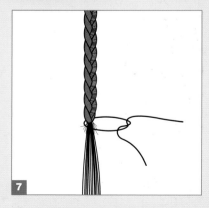

Two-Hand Twists (Double-Strand Twists)

1. This easiest of styles is done with natural hair. First determine how thick you want the twists to be. Begin by dividing one section of hair into two equal pieces.

2. Wrap the two pieces of the section around each other until you reach the ends.

3. Continue dividing the hair into sections and twisting until the entire head is complete.

BOMB TWIST

The bomb twist style is created with the same technique used for the two-hand twist, but special hair called bomb twist hair is added to the natural hair. The bomb twist hair is much softer than kinky twist hair (see pages 11 and 171, for example) and must be braided one to two inches, then tied before the twist can be started; otherwise, it will slip out. Refer to the instructions on page 6 for adding extensions to natural hair. For this style, it is very important that all the extension hair be the same length.

NUBE NUBE

The nube nube style is created with the same technique used for the two-hand twist, but curly human hair is added to the natural hair, which gives the style a wilder look. Refer to the instructions on page 6 for adding extensions to natural hair.

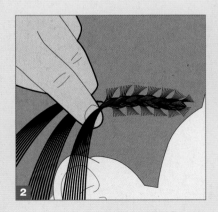

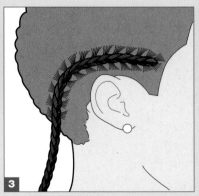

Cornrows

1. Begin by joining the synthetic or human hair to the natural hair, as described on page 7.

2. A cornrow is a section of hair that is braided flat to the scalp. To create this style, continue to braid the hair, but pick up and join natural hair to each section of synthetic hair as you create each link in the cornrow.

3. Continue to braid the hair into cornrows until you have reached the desired length.

Individual Braids

1. To create individual braids (individuals), begin by adding extensions for a braid as described on page 7.

2. Continue to braid the hair from roots to end until you've reached the desired length.

PIXIES

Pixies are created with the same technique used for individuals, but the strands are turned over as they are braided, and the braids are very tight, each link in the braid very close to the previous one. You can curl the ends to finish the style, tie them off with thread, or if you're using yarn or synthetic hair, you can seal the ends using a hot curling iron.

SPANISH WAVE

Spanish wave hair is joined to the natural hair as if individual braids were being created, but the braid is stopped after the end of the natural hair is reached, and the Spanish wave hair is left loose and twisted lightly to the ends.

The names that describe the types of hair used in this book may vary by brand. Where available, we have included a couple of different names for the same type of hair.

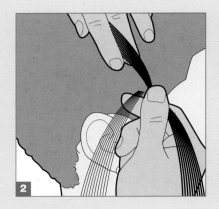

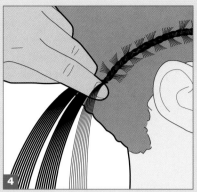

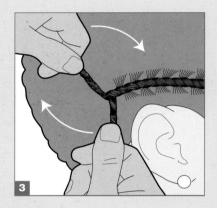

Senegalese Twist Cornrows

1. To create Senegalese twist cornrows, begin by adding extensions for a twist as described on page 6.

2. As you do with regular (braided) cornrows, pick up and join a small section of natural hair to each section of synthetic hair in the direction you want the cornrow to lie as you create each twist in the coil that forms the Senegalese twist cornrow.

3. Continue to coil the two twisted sections tightly around each other, carefully moving the hair in your left hand to your right hand, and vice versa. Be sure the twists and coils remain tight.

4. Continue steps 2 and 3 until the cornrow is the desired length. To finish, dip the ends into hot water to seal them.

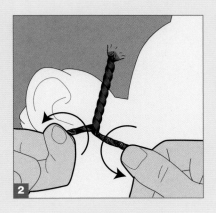

Senegalese Twists

1. To create Senegalese twists, begin by adding extensions for a twist as described on page 6.

2. Continue to twist the individual sections tightly, creating a ropelike effect. As you twist, tightly coil the two sections together until the Senegalese twist is the desired length.

3. To finish, dip the ends into hot water to seal them.

4. For a natural effect, you can fray the ends of the hair instead of sealing them with hot water. Bundle a few of the twists in your hand, holding the twists about two inches from the end. Using scissors or a blade, fray the ends of the hair, being sure to hold them away from both yourself and the person whose hair you are styling.

KINKY TWISTS

1. Use the same technique that's used for Senegalese twists, but use kinky hair and twist and coil the hair much more softly and loosely. You can also braid the hair extension hair in and then begin twisting.

2. To curl the ends of the hair, you can use rollers, or you can gather the ends into several large braids and dip them in hot water. Allow the ends to remain in the water for a few minutes, then remove the hair and take the braids out. The little crinkles at the ends of the twists provide the finishing touch.

NUBIAN TWISTS

Nubian twists are just like kinky twists, but synthetic Nubian hair is used. The hair comes already coiled in the twists, but to create the style, you must separate the strands, twist or braid them into the natural hair to anchor them, and then twist them together using the same technique that's used for kinky twists.

YARN TWISTS

Yarn twists are created just like Senegalese twists are, but yarn is used instead of synthetic or pony hair. To finish the twist, you must seal the ends with a hot curling iron.

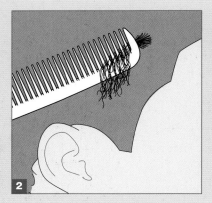

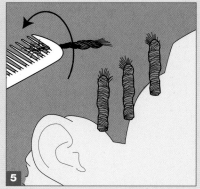

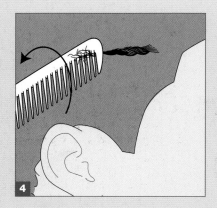

Gel Twists

1. Be sure you have a rattail comb (or any fine-tooth comb) and black gel to create this hairstyle. You can use the basic grid design shown on page 129, or you can create your own design.

2. Apply gel to a small piece of hair (one of the sections you've created). Comb through the hair to be sure that the gel coats the strands thoroughly.

3. Hook the comb into the hair so that the teeth of the comb are holding the hair next to the scalp.

4. Begin twisting the comb (left or right, your choice, but twist in the same direction for the entire style unless your design calls for a different technique).

5. Continue twisting the hair with the comb, simultaneously pulling the comb gently away from the scalp until you reach the end of the hair.

6. When the style is finished, the hair must be dried completely—either for about thirty minutes under a hair drier or by air drying.

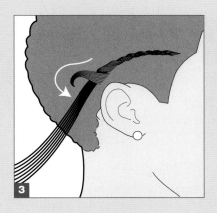

Flat Twists

In general, when you're creating a style with flat twists, you are working toward the centerpiece of the style; in our example, on page 63, the style culminates in a bun at the top of the wearer's head. Be sure to map out your design so that your twists will flow into your style centerpiece. This style, like gel twists, cannot be washed; if you wash out the gel, you'll wash out the hairstyle, too.

1. To begin, take the natural hair that's in the space where the bun will sit, and braid it up and into a bun.

2. Next attach a lock of synthetic hair to a section of the natural hair and apply gel to both.

3. To create the flat twist, turn the lock of hair over, almost as if you're turning a page in a book, a little at a time, picking up small sections of natural hair along the bottom of the twist and pulling them over the twist, incorporating them as you move along the head.

4. When you reach the bottom of the bun you created with the natural hair, continue to twist the hair (at this point you will not be incorporating more natural hair), and wrap it around the bun. Pin the twist in place. You can cut the synthetic hair (i.e., make the twists shorter) if the bun is too large or incorporate more synthetic hair (i.e., make the twists longer) if the bun is too small. To incorporate more synthetic hair into the twist, in your hand spread out the lock of synthetic hair you're already working with and lay the new hair on top of it, blending the strands of the two to create a single lock of hair.

The gel twist and flat twist hairstyles cannot be washed. Washing your hair will wash the gel—and the hairstyle—right out.

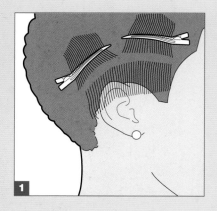

Invisible Cornrows

1. To begin, leave out about an inch of natural hair along the hairline, all the way around the head. This natural hair will be used as camouflage. It will be combed into the human hair to hide the place where the human hair is attached to the natural hair.

2. Next, part the natural hair into equal sections going from the front of the head straight to the back; this design will make the style look nice and full.

3. Join the human hair to the natural hair (see page 7 for instructions on joining extension hair to natural hair).

4. Begin to cornrow the human hair into the natural hair (see page 8 for instructions on braiding cornrows).

5. As you create the cornrows with the human hair and natural hair, pull the human hair out so that it is on top of the cornrows, hiding the cornrows.

6. Continue braiding the hair into cornrows until all the natural hair has been braided. Use the natural hair that you left out of the cornrows along the hairline (see step 1) to hide the cornrows along the outside of the head.

Kinky Long Length Human Hair

1. Braid the human hair into the natural hair from the scalp to about one inch out (see instructions on page 7 for attaching human hair to natural hair).

2. Tie a knot in the human hair at the point at which you stop braiding (about one inch from the scalp). Because human hair is comparatively soft and smooth, it will slip out if you don't tie or glue it in place.

3. Twist the hair softly and gently out to its ends.

Human Hair Lacing

1. Begin to braid the human hair into one small section of the natural hair, creating an individual braid. As you braid, pull the human hair out of the braid so that it hides the braid.

2. Continue this braid until all the natural hair has been braided. Allow the human hair to hang down naturally.

3. Continue this technique until you have completed braiding the human hair in all over the head.

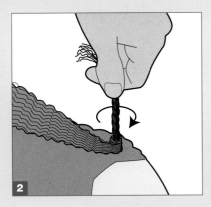

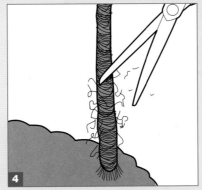

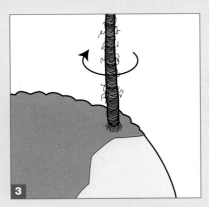

Dreadlock Extensions

1. Braid kinky human hair into natural hair for about two inches (see page 7). Let the rest of the hair extension hang loose.

2. Return to the scalp, where you began the braid, and begin wrapping the braid with a long strand of kinky human hair (the same type of hair you've braided into the natural hair). Wrap the hair tightly; you must completely hide the braid and the rest of the attached lock of hair.

3. Continue wrapping until you have reached the end of the attached lock of hair.

4. Finish the dread by rolling the last three inches or so between your palms for several minutes. Carefully trim any broken hairs along the length of the dread with scissors.

SILKY DREADS

Create silky dreads just as you create regular dreads, but use synthetic hair instead of human hair to wrap the dreads for this shinier look.

FAA-LING-YING

Create the faa-ling-ying style just as you created regular dreads, but use thread instead of human hair to wrap the dreads for this dramatic look.

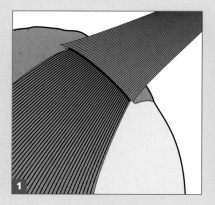

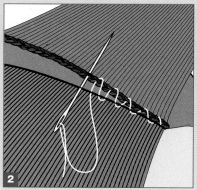

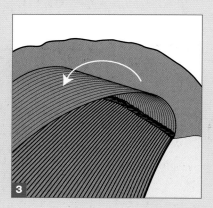

Weaves

1. Cornrow the natural hair, either in a spiral beginning at the back of the neck, or from front to back from the forehead to the crown and from side to side from the crown to the neckline. If you cornrow the natural hair from front to back in the front of the head, you must leave out a section of natural hair at the center front of the head to cover the tracks at the top of the head (see steps 3 and 4).

2. Weave hair comes in "tracks," or large sections of hair with a band that's used to attach the weave to the natural hair. With a needle and thread that matches the color of the weave, sew the tracks onto the cornrows.

3. For hair that is styled in cornrows from front to back, comb the natural hair that was left out with a straightening comb, so that it matches the added hair, and part it to cover the tracks to the left and right.

4. Comb the natural hair into the weave hair to integrate the two.

5. Style as desired. Human hair weaves can be washed normally.

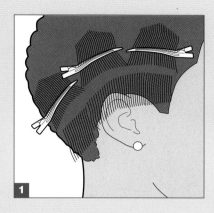

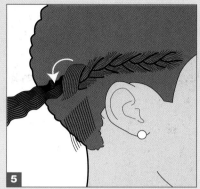

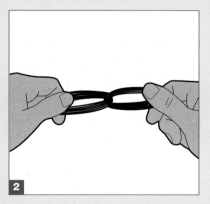

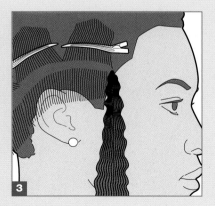

Goddess Braids

1. To create a goddess braid from scratch, begin by parting the natural hair into sections. The number of sections should be the same as the number of goddess braids you plan to create. As always, the hair you are not working on should be clipped or braided so that it's out of the way.

2. Crisscross two lengths of synthetic hair. In both hands, hold the two sides together, so you have a total of two strands.

3. Hold the synthetic hair at the hairline, perpendicular to one section of natural hair.

4. With your index finger, take a small piece of the natural hair and join it to the synthetic hair.

5. Braid the joined natural and synthetic hair inward (overhand; the opposite of how cornrows are braided), continuing to pick up and join natural hair to the synthetic hair.

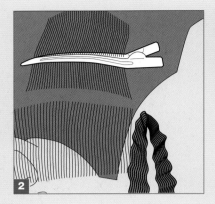

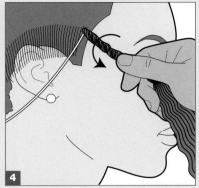

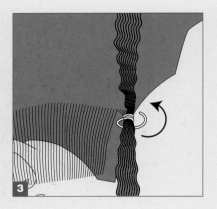

African Twists

This exotic-looking style lasts about six weeks, but be warned: it hurts—the hair is twisted and pulled very tightly.

1. Before you begin, have at hand synthetic hair and thread that matches the color of the synthetic hair.

2. Begin by joining the synthetic hair to the natural hair, holding the center point of the synthetic hair next to the section of the hair you're working on.

3. Wrap the thread around the synthetic and natural hair four or five times to anchor the synthetic hair, and then fold the synthetic hair in half so you are holding the natural hair and all the synthetic hair in one large lock.

4. Twist the synthetic hair between your thumb and fingers for about five or six inches.

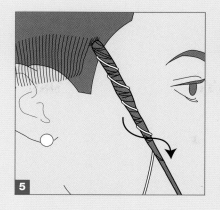

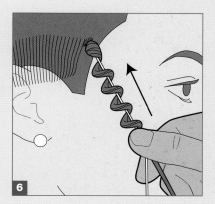

5. Wrap the thread at an angle around the twisted synthetic hair for about three inches.

6. Push the hair up the thread, simultaneously pulling the thread away from the head, so that the hair is coiled tightly around the thread. Be sure to hold the synthetic hair tightly so the twist does not come undone.

7. Repeat steps 4 through 6 until you have reached the desired length. You can add more synthetic hair into the existing hair if you want a longer twist. To do this, spread out the loose hair that you have in your hand, and lay the additional hair on top of it, blending the two into one lock. Continue twisting and wrapping as usual.

8. Repeat steps 4 through 6 until you have reached the desired length.

9. Wrap the thread about ten times around the tip of the twist and tie a double knot in it. Cut the ends of the thread and the ends of the hair. Carefully trim any broken hairs along the length of the twist with scissors.

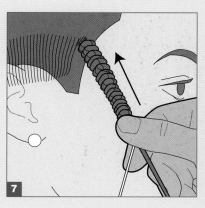

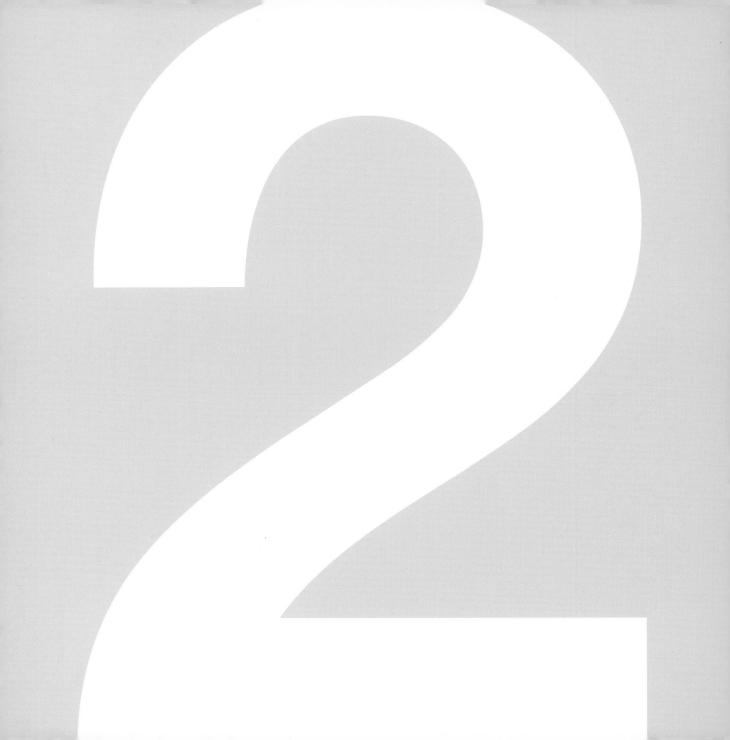

HAIRSTYLES CREATED WITH SYNTHETIC HAIR

Cornrows are a common style, worn by men, women, and children alike, but there are many ways to part, position, and finish the style to make one look different from all others. Cornrows can be left in for about a month. After that, every-day wear and tear will cause them to look rough.

Feeding Cornrows

The top layer of this style (from forehead to crown) shows alternating larger and smaller feeding cornrows. To create feeding cornrows, follow the instructions for cornrows on page 8, but continue to feed more synthetic hair into the cornrow as you braid, so that the cornrow becomes thicker as it becomes longer.

The bottom layer of this style is micro individuals (very small individual braids).

The blond ends of all the braids are left loose and straight.

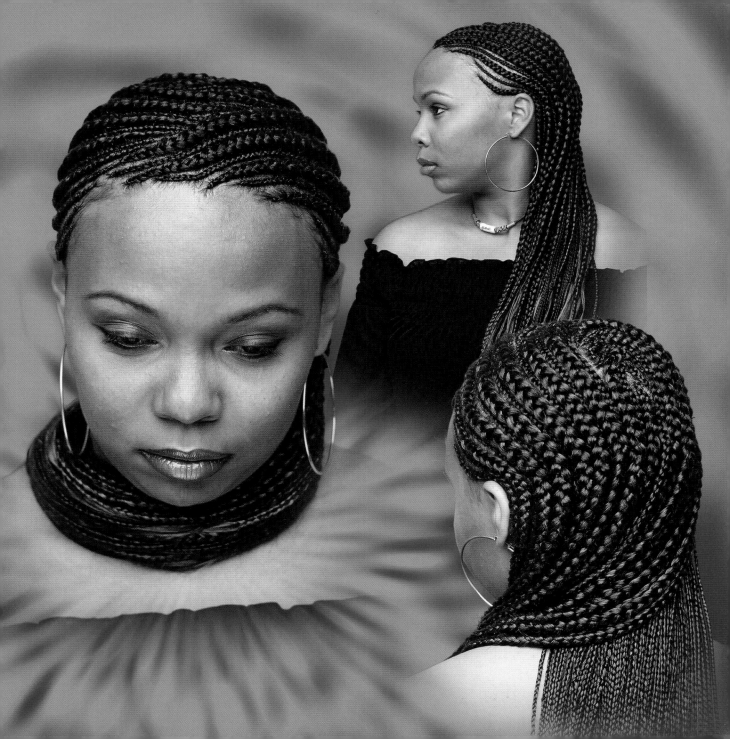

CORNROWS

Individual Braids Styled in Cornrows

The left-hand and bottom photos show individual braids begun in the front, then transitioned at the ear line to cornrows, and then transitioned back to individuals at the base of the head. To finish the look, the red ends of the pony hair are left loose and straight. As you can see, even after braiding is complete, long hair like this allows the wearer many styling options.

Cornrows and Individuals

The top and right-hand photos show cornrows created with pony hair in the front. At the crown of the head, the ends of the cornrows are left loose, and individual braids are created at the back of the head.

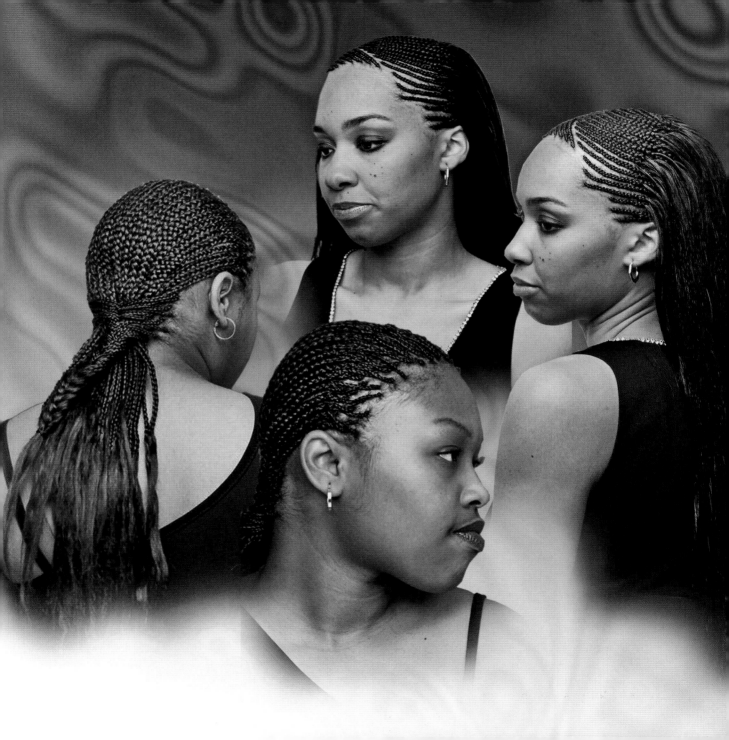

Coiled Cornrows and Individuals

In this style, using synthetic hair, the front is styled in cornrows to the crown of the head. At the crown of the head, the hair from the cornrows is simply plaited to the end, and then groups of five or six of these plaits are coiled and pinned in sections at the crown. The back hair is braided into individuals and left to hang loose.

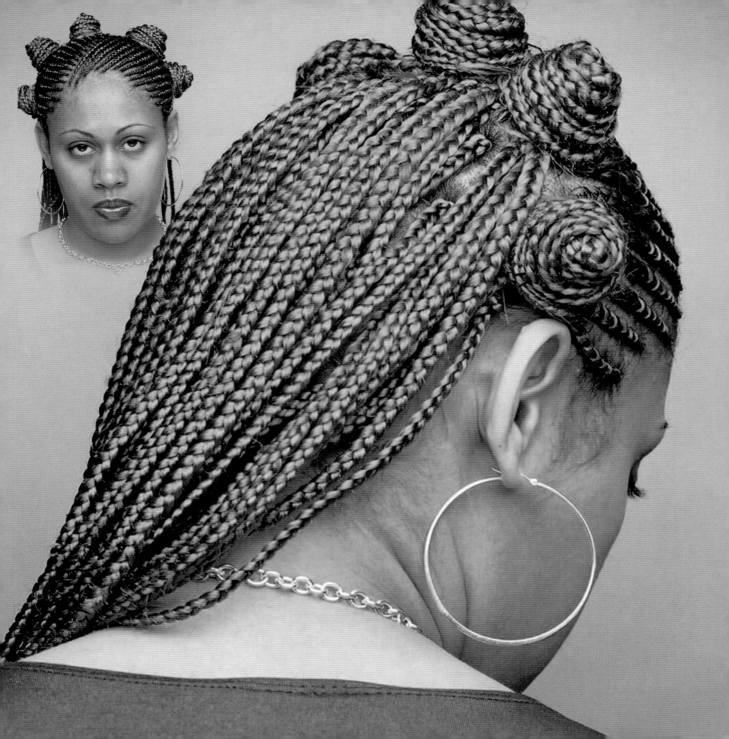

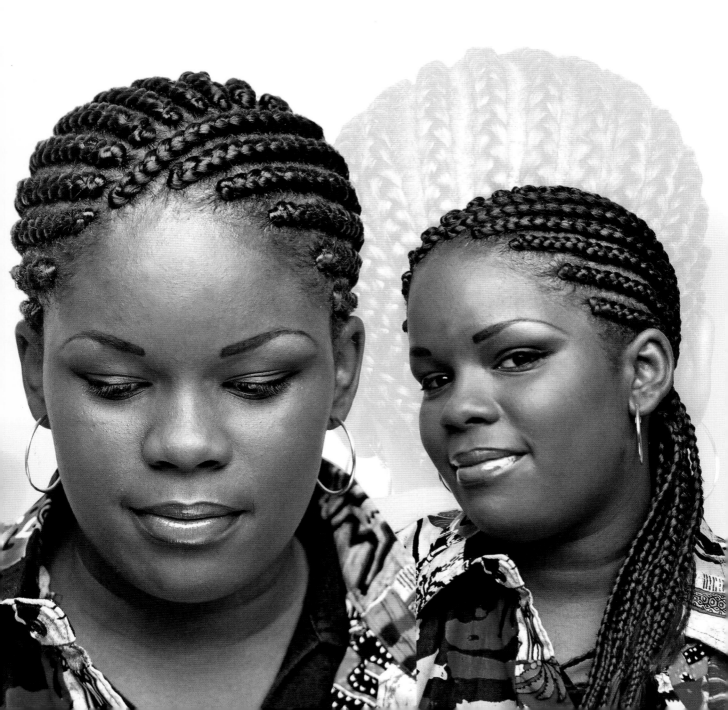

One-Layer Cornrows

In this style, simple, large, one-layer cornrows are created with synthetic hair from the front of the head to the neckline. In the left-hand photo, the plaits are pulled into a bun; on the right, the plaits are loose. The ends of the braids are left loose.

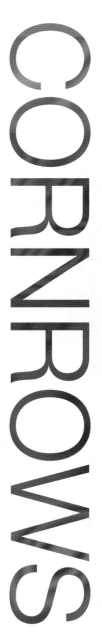

CORNROWS

Multilayer Cornrows

To create multilayer cornrows like these, begin creating cornrows with synthetic hair at the front of the head. When you reach the crown, discontinue the cornrows and simply braid the rest of that hair out to the end. Clip those braids out of the way and then create cornrows down from the crown to the base of the head. When you reach the neckline, braid the rest of the hair out to the end, finishing with the ends of the braids loose and straight.

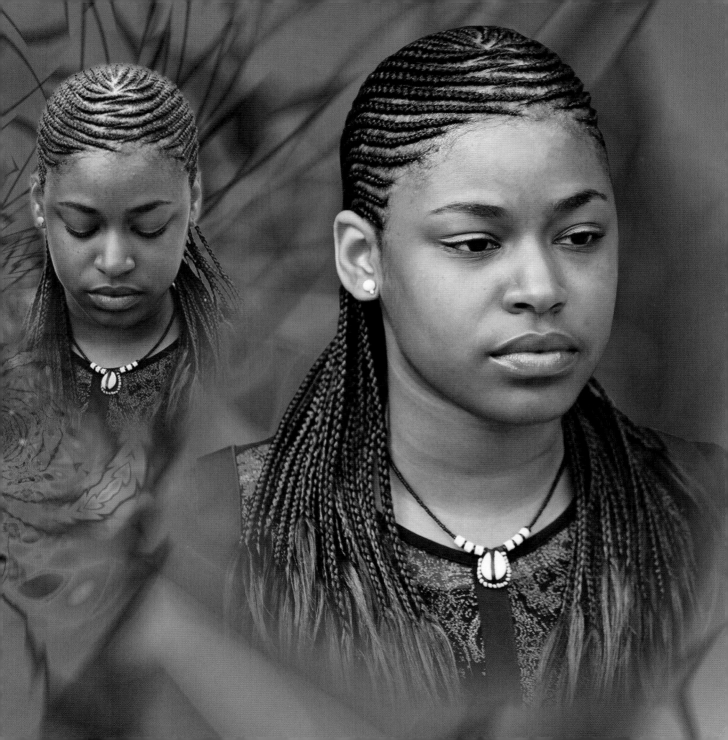

Multilayer Cornrows

In this technique, the hair is styled in cornrows for a few inches and then braided individually to the end, leaving the blond tips of the two-tone pony hair curled and loose.

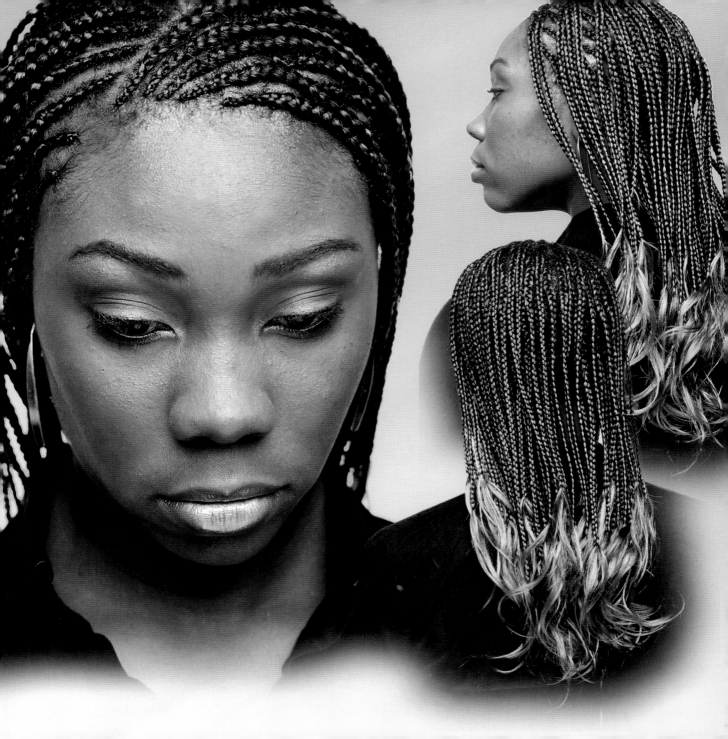

CORNROWS

One-Layer Crazy Cornrows

The "crazy" in "crazy cornrows" just means that different sizes of cornrows are used. These cornrows, made with pony hair, are spaced loosely, in contrast to those on the next page, which are very close together.

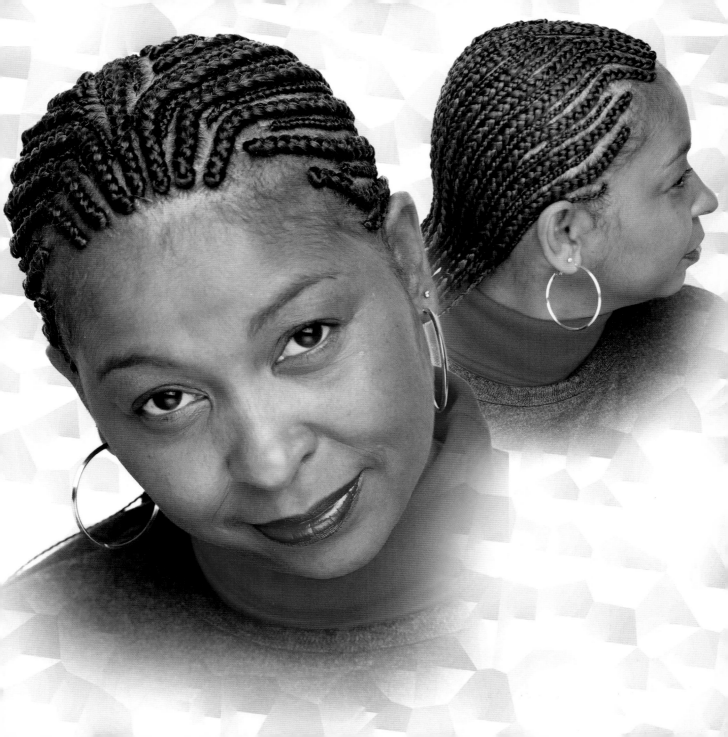

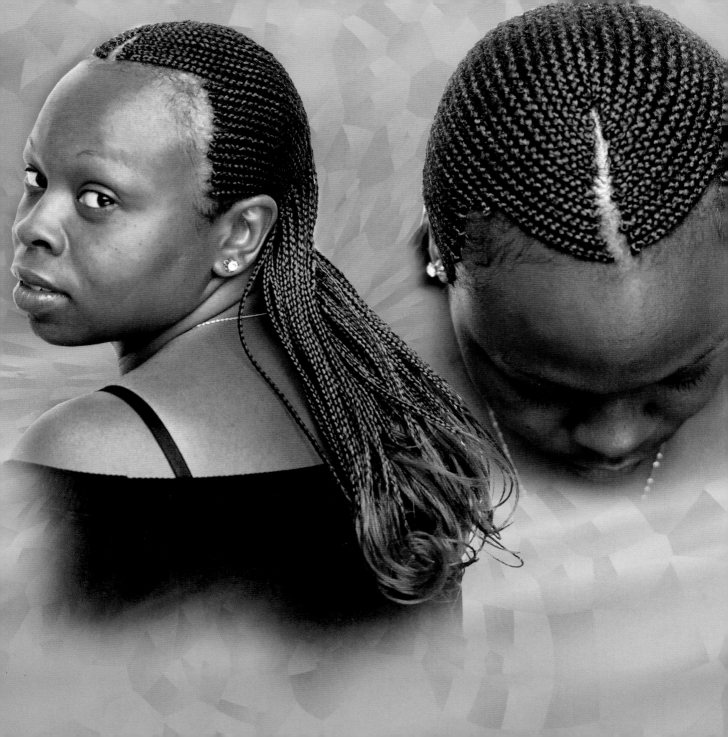

One-Layer Cornrows

In this style, a part is made at the center front, and the pony-hair cornrows are created in soft curves following the shape of the head. The ends of the braids are left loose and curled. The look is sleek and clean.

CORNROWS

Senegalese Twist Cornrows

These Senegalese twist cornrows, made with pony hair, are pulled back into a bun, and the ends are allowed to hang down in a ponytail. The ends of the braids are curled to finish the look. To create Senegalese twist cornrows, see the step-by-step instructions on page 10.

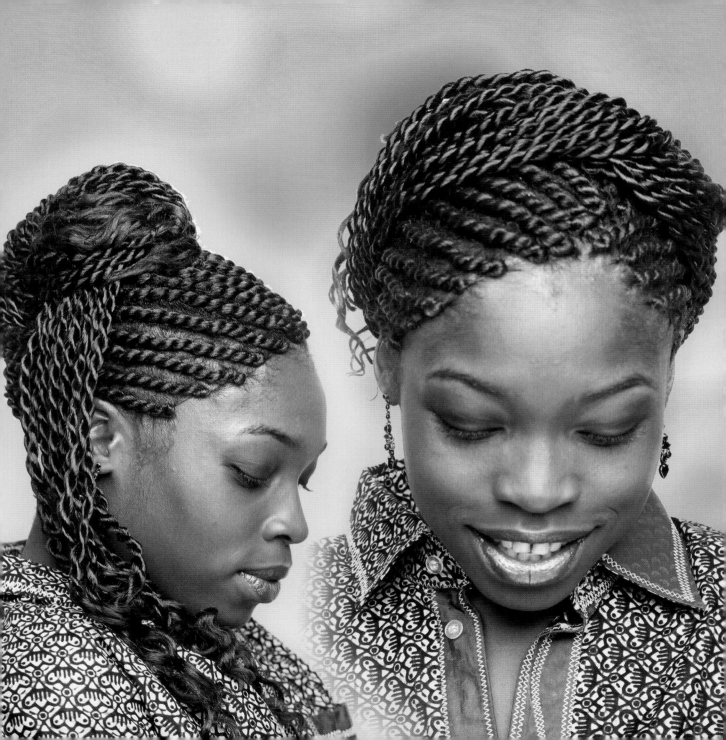

CORNROWS

Cornrows

This cornrow look is similar to the one on page 36, but here the hair is parted differently for a more geometric look in front, the cornrows are slightly larger and more widely spaced, and the ends of the braids are left to hang straight rather than curled.

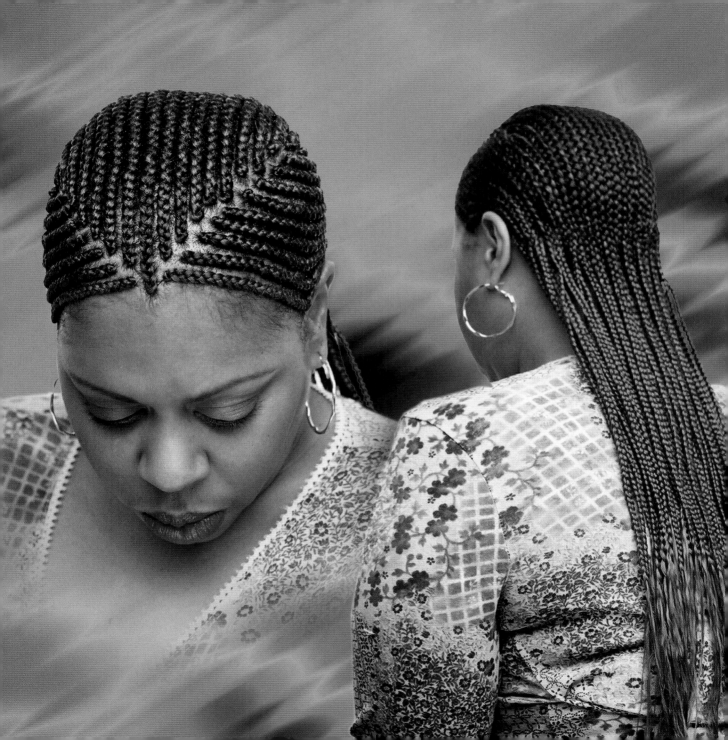

Individuals are a versatile hairstyle. They can be worn loose, pulled back into a ponytail or bun, coiled, or pinned back with clips or barrettes, allowing you the flexibility to create casual or formal styles. To create individuals, follow the step-by-step instructions on page 9. Individuals can usually be left in for about two months before they begin to show their age.

Individuals with the Ends Out

In the style shown here, the braids, made with straight pony hair, are finished at varying levels for a less uniform look, but all the ends are loose and straight. In the center and right-hand photos, the braids are allowed to hang loose for a relaxed, natural look. In the left-hand photo, the braids in the front are pulled to one side to frame the face, the rest of the braids are pulled up into a ponytail at the crown of the head, and the ponytail is held with an additional piece of the same hair used to create the individuals.

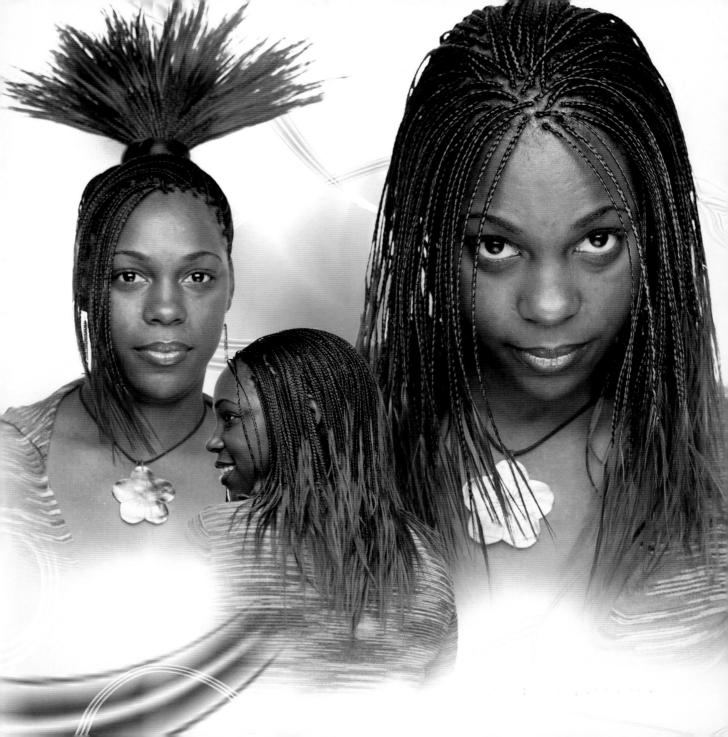

Individuals with the Ends Out

In the style shown here, individuals, created with synthetic hair, are made larger and closer together for a fuller effect. The ends are allowed to hang loose and straight. At center, a few braids in front frame the face and the rest are pulled back into a high ponytail. At left and right, the braids are left out for a natural, relaxed look.

Caring for Your Hair

To wash individuals and Senegalese hair styles:
1. Turn warm water on low.
2. Wet hair thoroughly.
3. Apply shampoo generously and work through hair.
4. Gently run your fingers through the hair. Remember, this is not your natural hair. If you are not gentle, you may end up with a handful of hair.
5. Rinse thoroughly and repeat.
6. Apply conditioner carefully.
7. Rinse well.
8. Towel dry.
9. Air dry or use a hair drier to finish drying your hair.

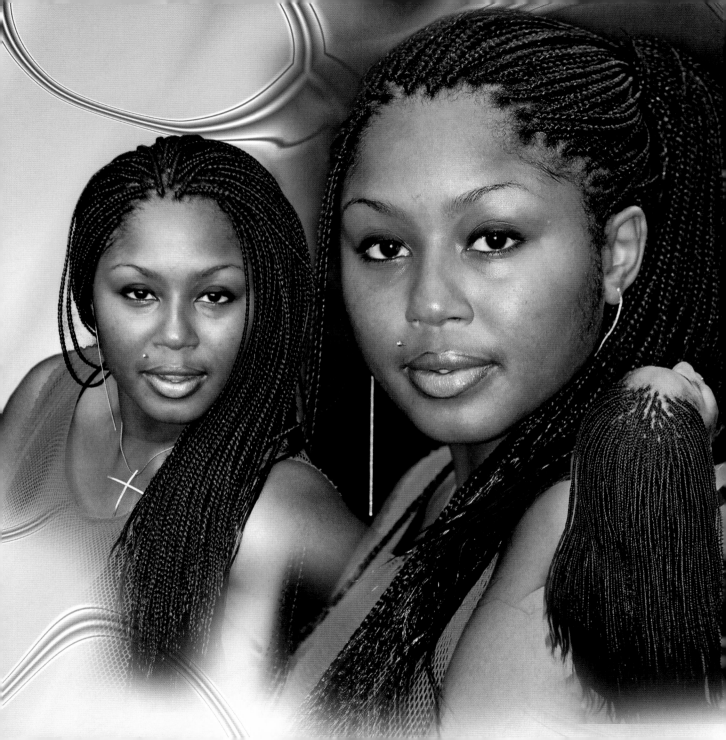

Individuals with Straight Ends

The left-hand photos show the front and rear views of individual braids with the ends out. Both burgundy and black synthetic hair is used, which demonstrates the variety of looks you can achieve even with this basic style. In the top photo, some braids are left out to frame the face, and the rest of the front braids are pulled into a high ponytail and wrapped with a few braids, resulting in a natural, organic look.

The right-hand and center photos show several views of individual braids, but in this instance, the braids are large (also known as "big box braids"), very long, and made with all black synthetic hair. At bottom right, the braids are worn loose, and the center and top right photos show the braids loosely pulled back into a high ponytail, again with braids wrapping around the base.

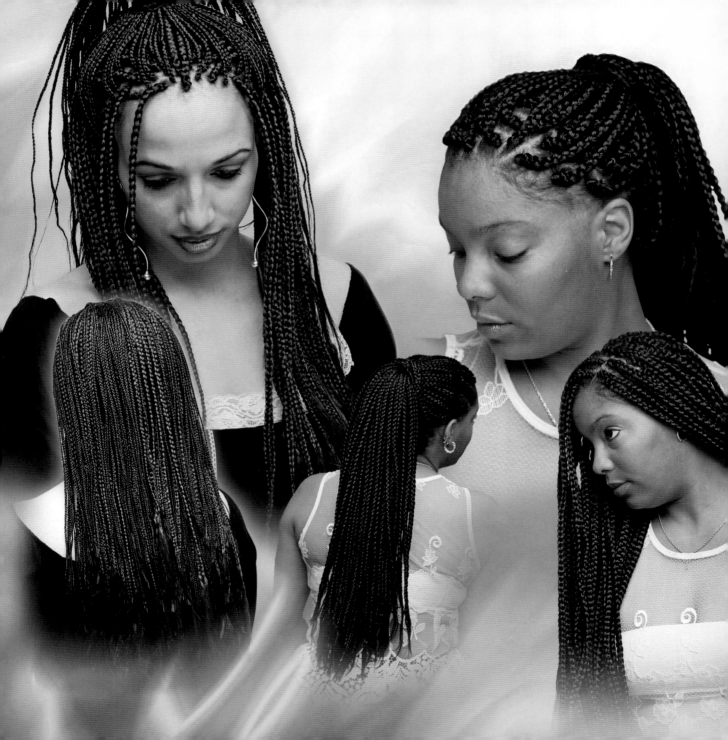

Mixed Individuals and Senegalese Twists

Another way to create a distinctive look is to combine braid types. These three photos show a combination of individual Senegalese braids in burgundy and individual braids in black, all made with synthetic hair. The style is finished with the ends loose and straight. In the right-hand photo all the braids are pulled back into a high ponytail, just one of the options for varying this style.

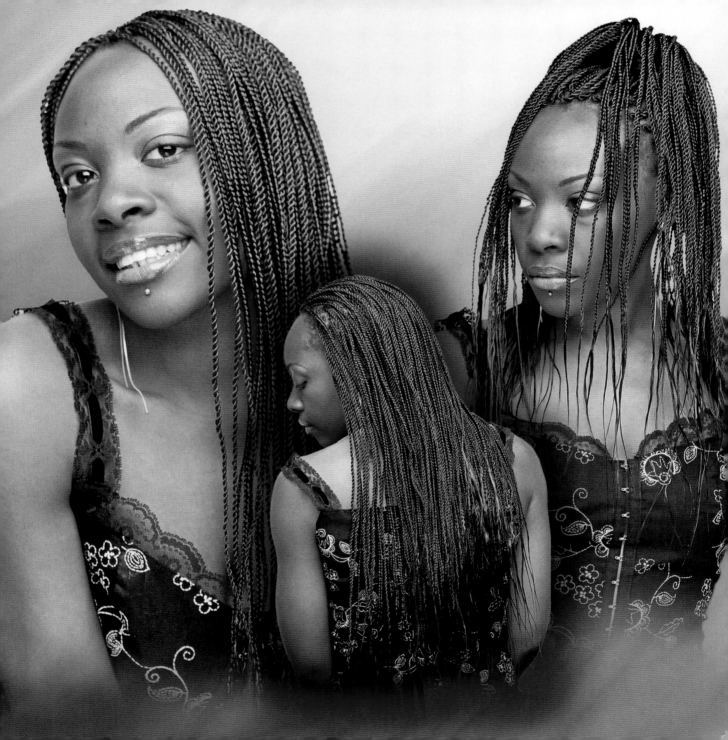

Layered Hair Individually Braided

To add some volume, the individuals in this style are of varying lengths. The blond ends are curled softly to complete this romantic look. In the center photo, the front braids are pulled back into a bun on the crown of the head, and the ends of the braids lie across the front of the head and onto the forehead for a face-framing look suitable for a night out.

tip

To create a layered hairstyle, be sure that the hair you are adding, whether it's human, pony, or synthetic, is all the same length. Naturally, where the hair is attached to the head will determine how long it appears to be. In other words, hair that you attach to the top of the head will not hang down as far as hair that you attach closer to the hairline.

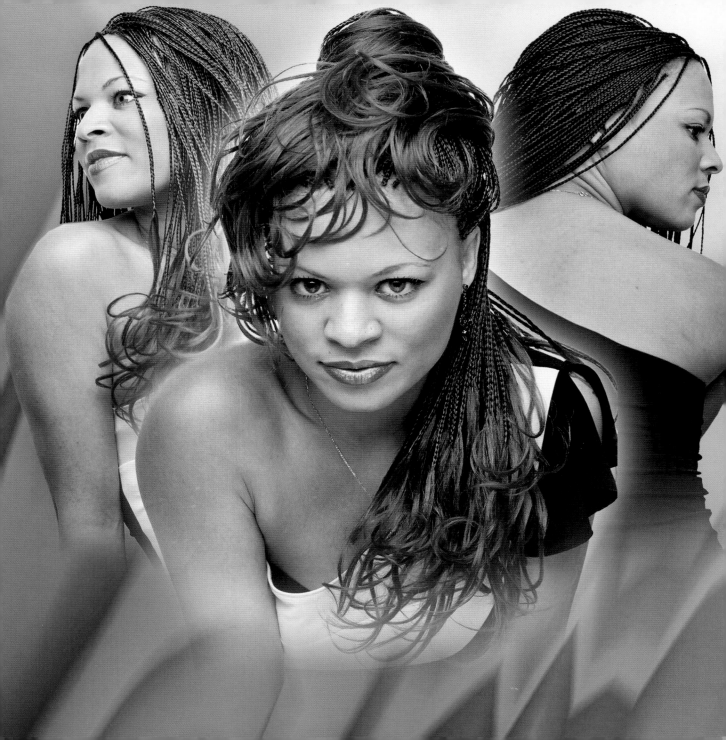

Twists are created the same way Senegalese braids are, but the hair is not held as tightly or twisted as tightly, so the result is a looser, softer look. Twists can usually be left in for about two months before they start to look worn—but by then you'll probably be ready for a new style anyway!

Twists

Here are two different lengths of twists, both created with kinky synthetic hair. In the center and upper right-hand photos, some of the twists are pulled back into a loose, high ponytail with some twists left down in front to frame the face and in back for a casual look.

TWISTS

tip

To finish twists, whether long or short, you can either leave them loose or dip the ends in hot water and curl them.

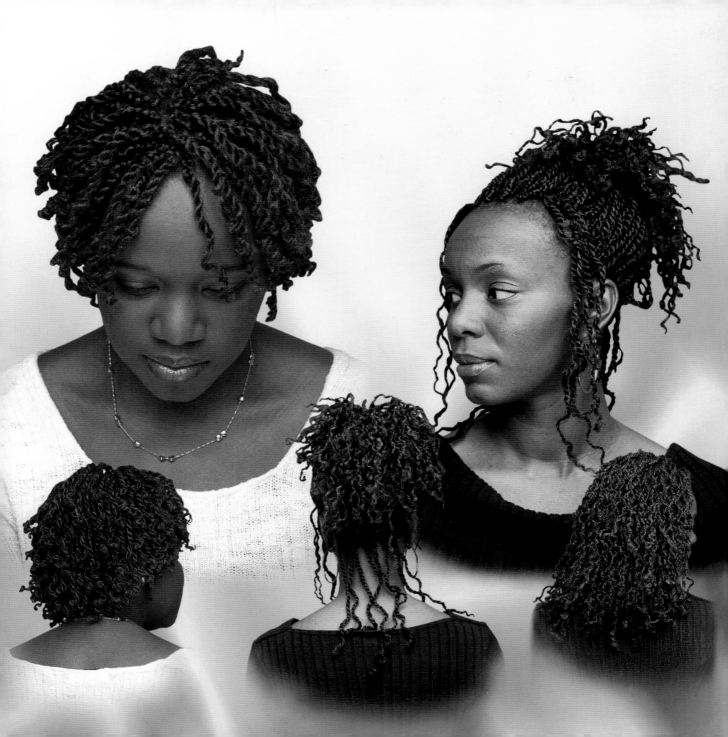

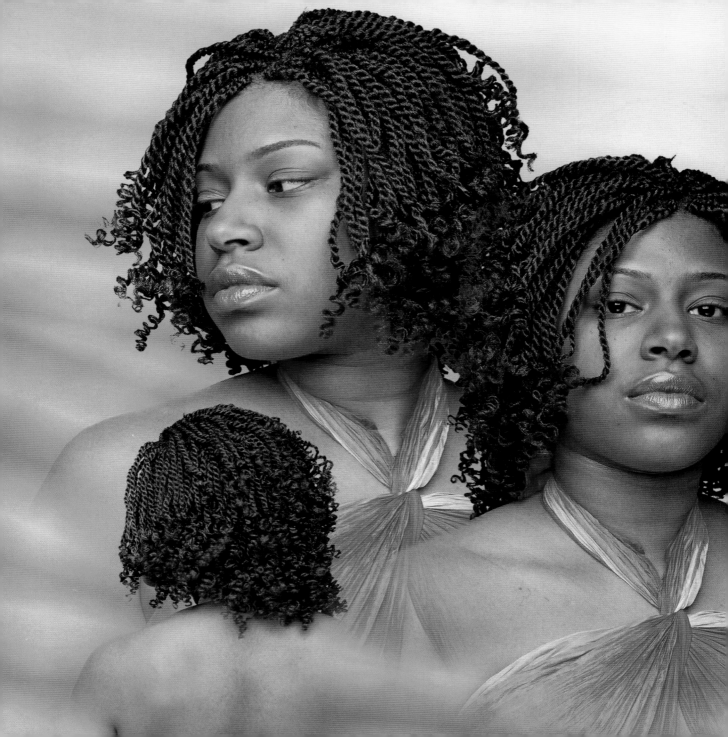

Medium-Length Twists

Twists offer great freedom for their wearer. You can work out and even swim with twists, and they stand up to everything the weather can throw at you. To a point, the older this style gets, the better it looks!

tip

Remember that for all styles in which you add synthetic or human hair to natural hair, you must begin by braiding or twisting the added hair into the natural hair tightly to ensure that it stays in place.

TWISTS

Nubian Twists—Long

Nubian twists are made with synthetic Nubian hair. The hair comes coiled, but to create the style, you must separate the strands, braid them into the natural hair to anchor them, and then twist them together again for the final look. On the left, the front twists are pulled up into a ponytail. On the right, the twists hang loose.

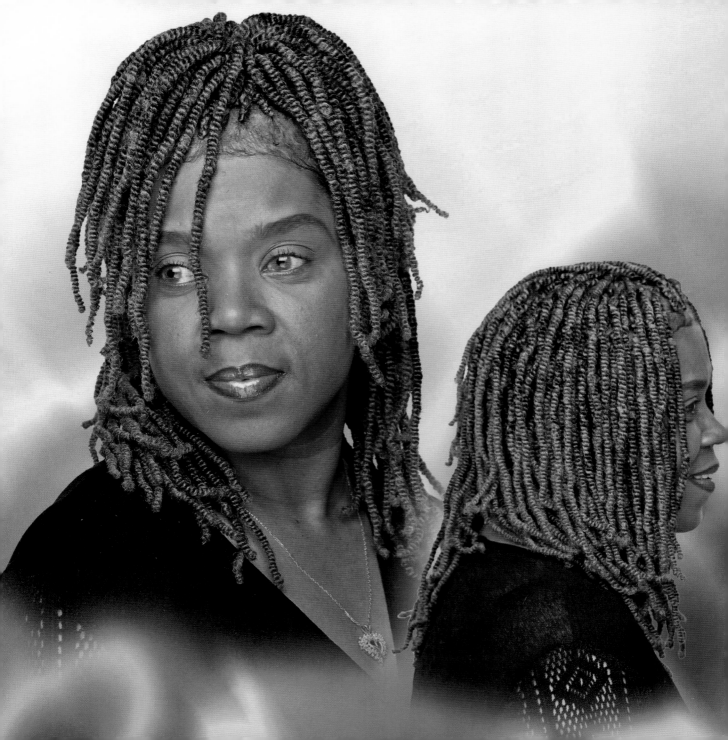

TWISTS

Nubian Twists—Short

For this layered style, two-tone black and burgundy synthetic Nubian hair is anchored to the natural hair with a few inches of braiding, then twisted into the final style. To create a layered style (in which all the ends do not fall to the same length), use synthetic hair pieces that are all the same length. As you braid the synthetic hair into the natural hair, the different positions it falls in on the head will determine how long it appears to be in the final style (hair attached to the bottom of the head will fall lower than that attached to the top of the head).

The hair used for most of the short styles in this book actually comes on a track (used for weaving) and is cut off to create these styles.

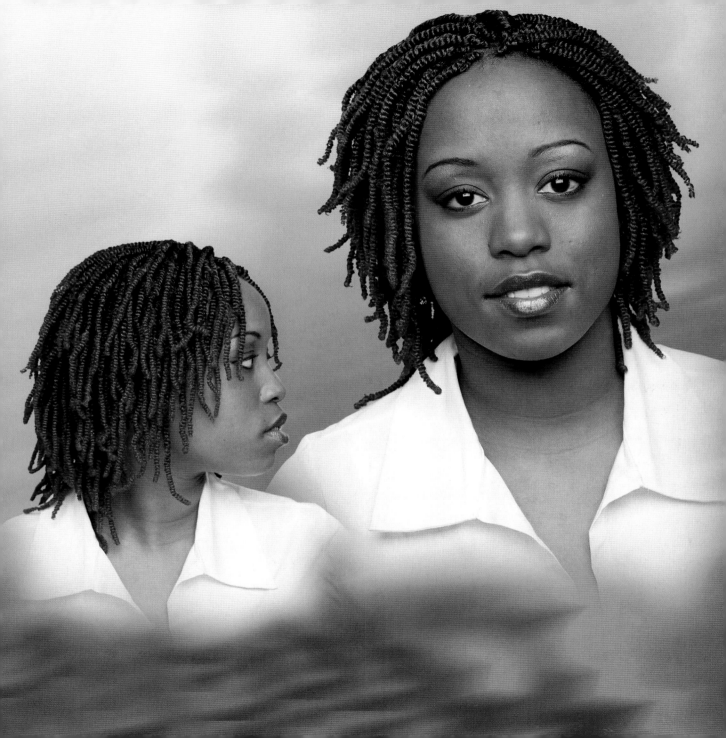

TWISTS

Bomb Twists

The synthetic hair used for bomb twists is softer and smoother than that used for kinky twists (page 171), for example. After it's braided into the natural hair, it must be tied as well; otherwise, you'll run the risk of it slipping out. To create the bomb twist, use the same technique as for the two-hand (double-strand) twist (page 8).

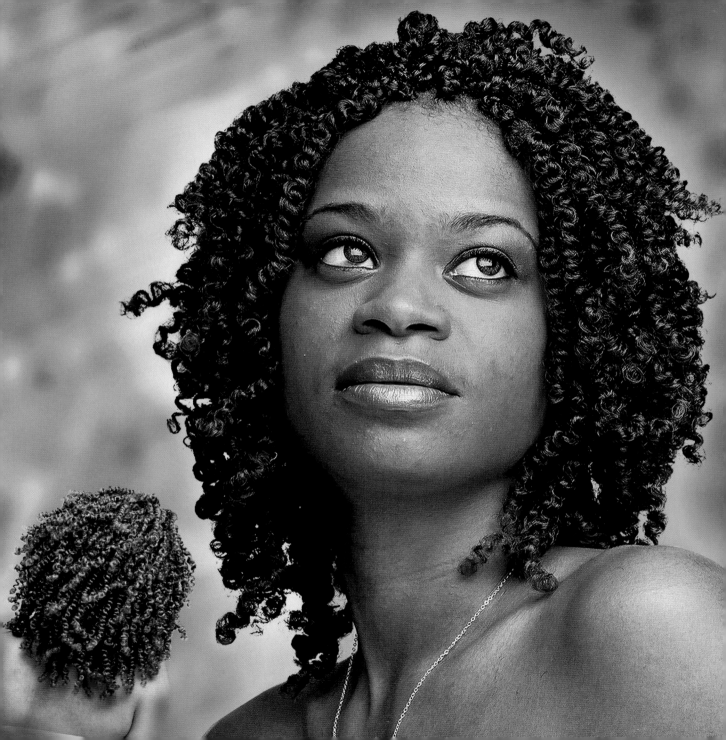

TWISTS

Flat Twists

The centerpiece of this gelled style is the bun, toward which all the flat twists are directed. The design for this style must be mapped out carefully, as all the twists must flow seamlessly toward the bun for the finished piece to look professional and stylish. Like the gel twist style, the flat twist style cannot be washed; if you wash your hair, you'll wash out the gel and the style too. You can, however, add ornaments, such as jeweled hairpins, to dress up this style. See page 13 for step-by-step instructions on how to create this style.

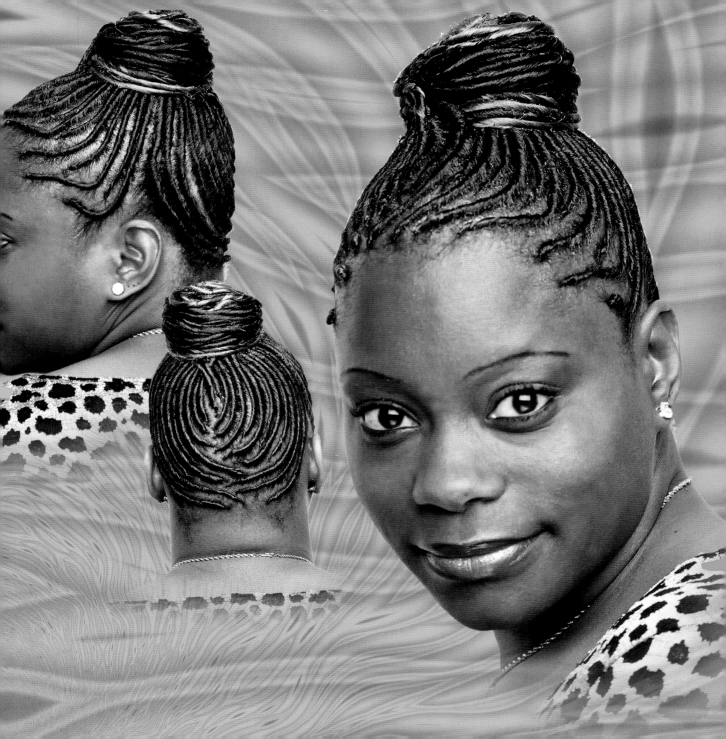

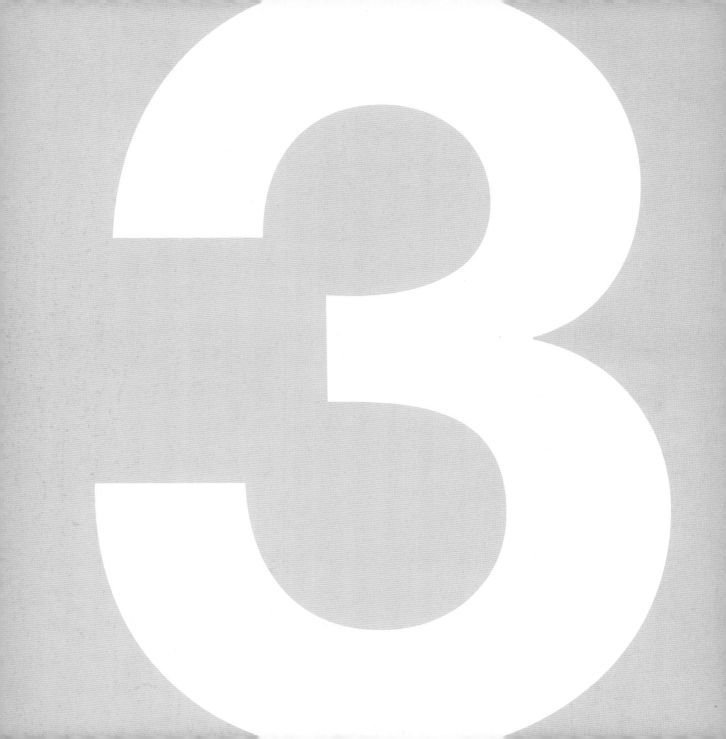

HAIRSTYLES CREATED WITH HUMAN HAIR

CORNROWS

Cornrows made with human hair, just like those made with synthetic hair, can usually be left in for about a month before everyday wear and tear causes them to show their age. And just like those made with synthetic hair, cornrows made with human hair can be designed in many different ways to showcase your individual style.

Three-Layer Cornrows

Very long wet and wavy human hair is used for this style. The first (bottom) layer is individuals; the second and third layers are cornrows; the long ends are left loose, full, and wavy.

Wet and wavy hair right out of the package is slightly wavy. After you attach it to the natural hair, wet it, then dry it. When it dries, it will be wavy, as shown in this finished style.

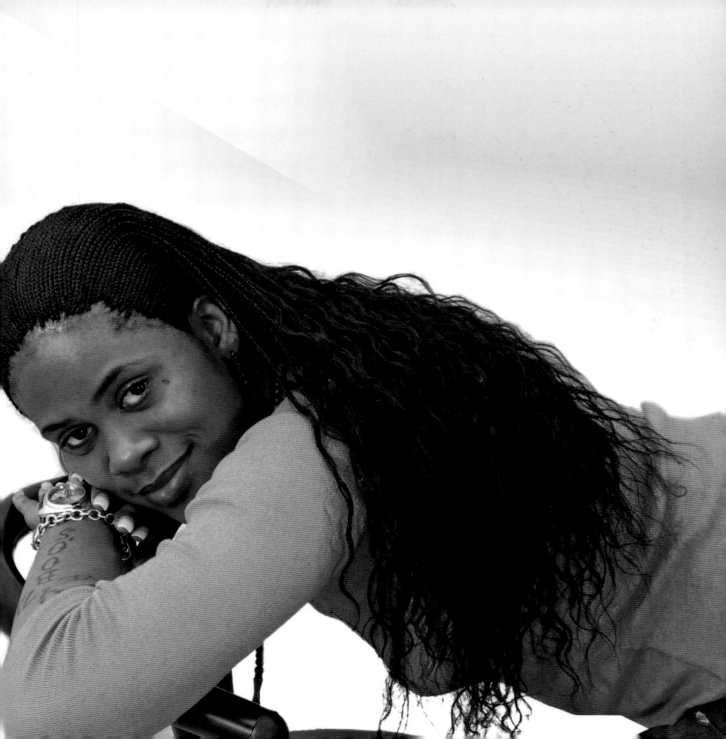

CORNROWS

Cornrows

For this style, long wet and wavy human hair is styled in cornrows beginning at the hairline, in toward the top of the head, back at an angle from the forehead, and up from both sides to the angled line from the top of the ear to the crown of the head, as shown in the photo on the right. When the cornrows meet at the top of the head, they are braided out, leaving a good length loose and wavy at the end. The back of the head is braided straight back in cornrows. When the style is complete, it can be worn out, as shown in the left-hand photo, or the cornrow braids can be gathered into one large braid at the top of the head, with the ends again left loose.

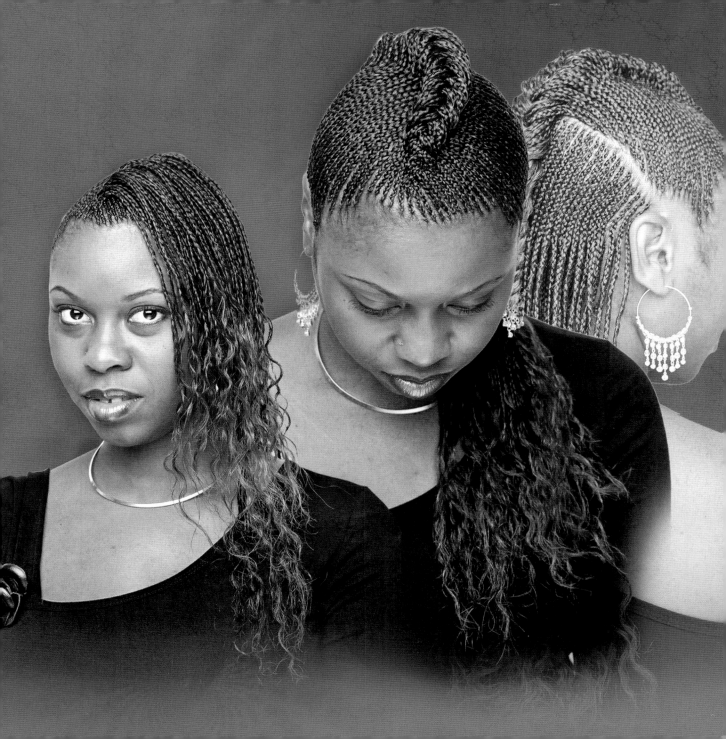

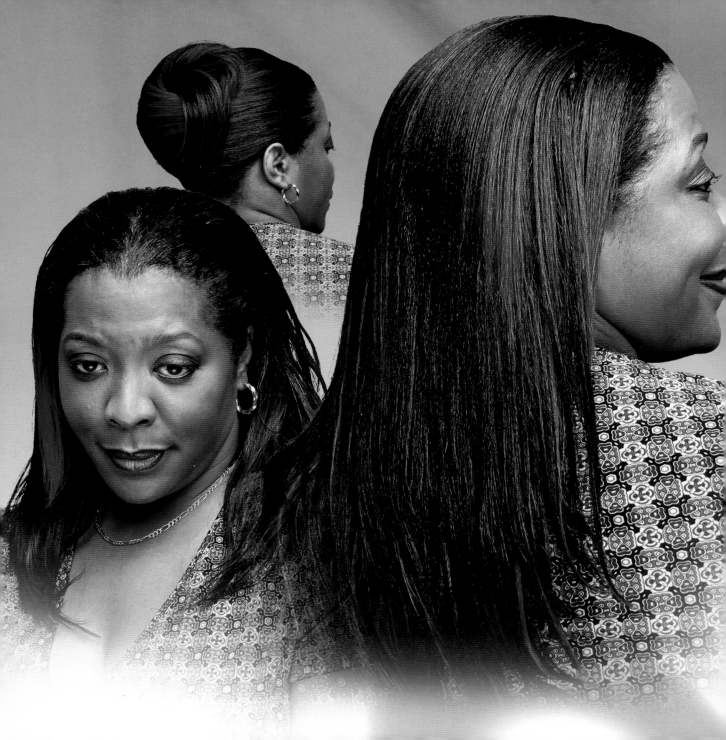

Invisible Cornrows

When this hairstyle is complete, the hair will look like a weave. (Refer to the step-by-step instructions on page 14 to learn how to create this hairstyle.) At top left the hair, black highlighted with burgundy, is pulled into a modified French twist. In the other two images, the hair is left down. The right-hand photo shows the angled layers, created after all the hair has been attached.

CORNROWS

You can usually wear your twists for about two months before they start to show their age, but some of the styles look great for three months or more.

Long, Full Twists

The style on the left is long two-tone twists created with kinky human hair, shown loose and free at top and bottom right. For a more formal look, the twists are piled at the back of the head at bottom left, with the front section left out to frame the face. On the right are one-color twists, again using kinky human hair, left loose at the top and pulled back in a dramatic style at bottom.

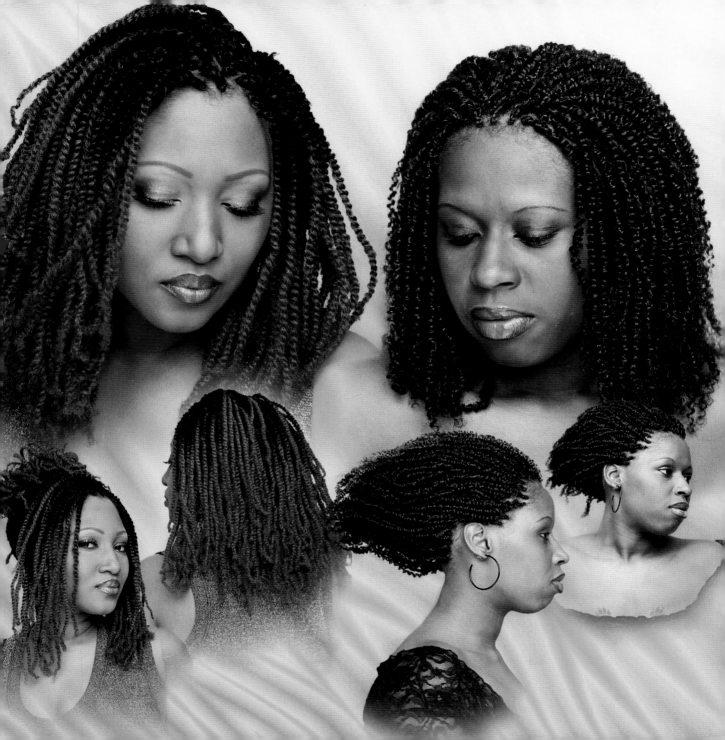

TWISTS

Nube Nube—Short

The nube nube hairstyle is created the same way two-hand twists are, in this case using corkscrew human hair that was cut off a weave track. This short nube nube hairstyle, created with curly black hair with red tips, still looked great even after three months.

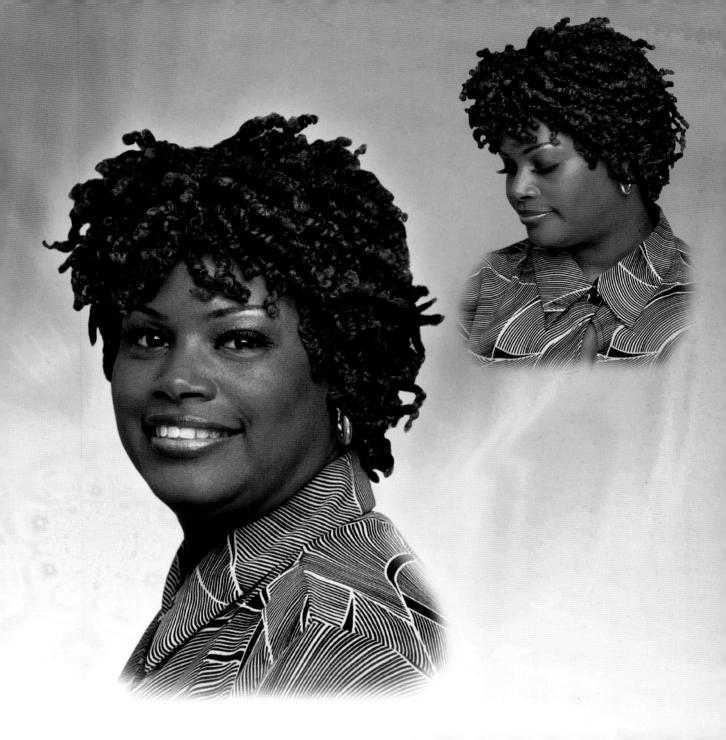

TWISTS

Nube Nube—Long

In these photos the nube nube hairstyle is illustrated in a much longer length, using one-color Bohemian human hair. The style is shown loose here but can be pulled back or up for different looks.

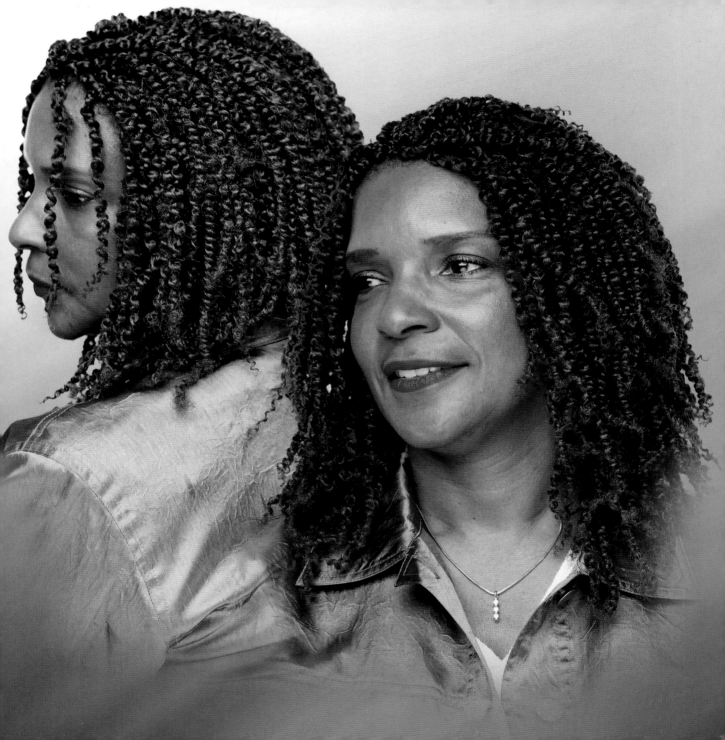

TWISTS

Nube Nube—Short

Though the style is the same, you can create very different looks with the

nube nube, as can be seen from the images on this page and the previous

two pages. Here the styles are made with Bohemian hair cut off a weave track.

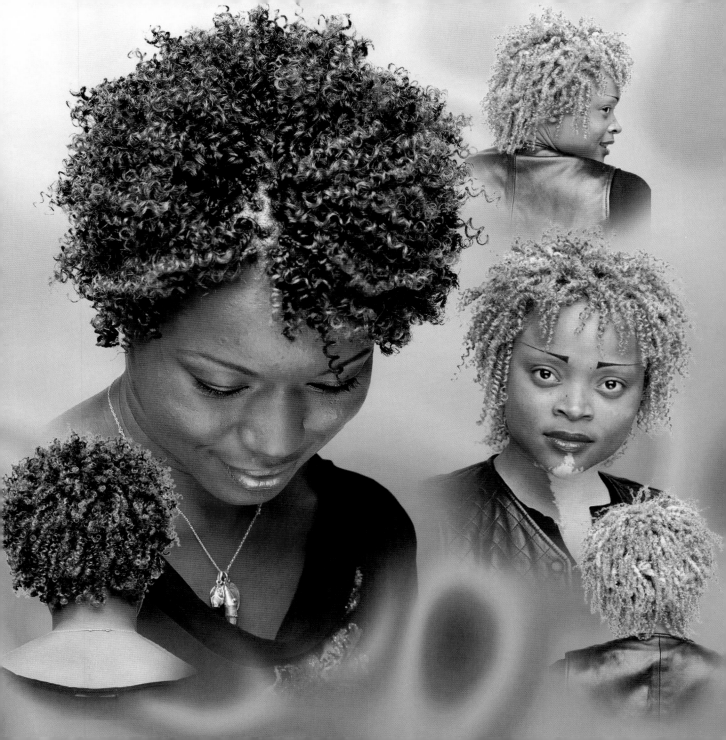

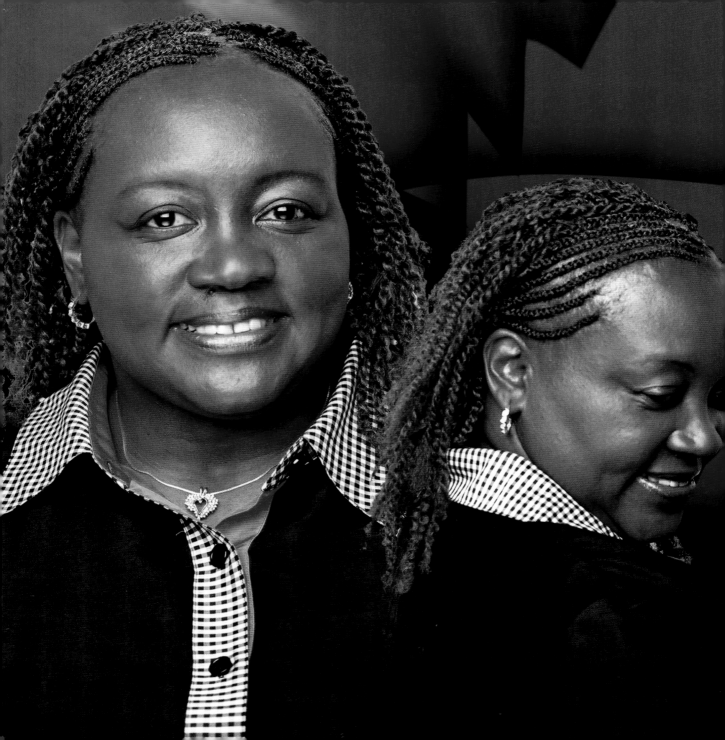

Cornrows with
Individual Nube Nube

In the photos shown here, the human hair, called Bohemian, is styled in just a few

cornrows in the front and individual nube nube in the back. See the step-by-step

instructions for cornrows on page 8. Nube nube are created the same way two-

handed twists are; see page 8 for step-by-step instructions.

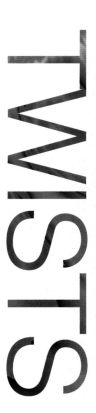

For individual braids with human hair, you must braid the human hair into the natural hair past the point where the natural hair ends, then either tie or glue (using nail glue) the human hair so it can't slip out. These styles usually last two months before you'll need to make a trip back to the salon for a new style.

Long Individuals

For this style, using Spanish perm wave hair, the braids are continued for just a short length, and the rest of the hair is allowed to fall loose, for a full, natural look. At bottom right, the hair is styled in a French twist, with the ends left loose for a slightly softer look.

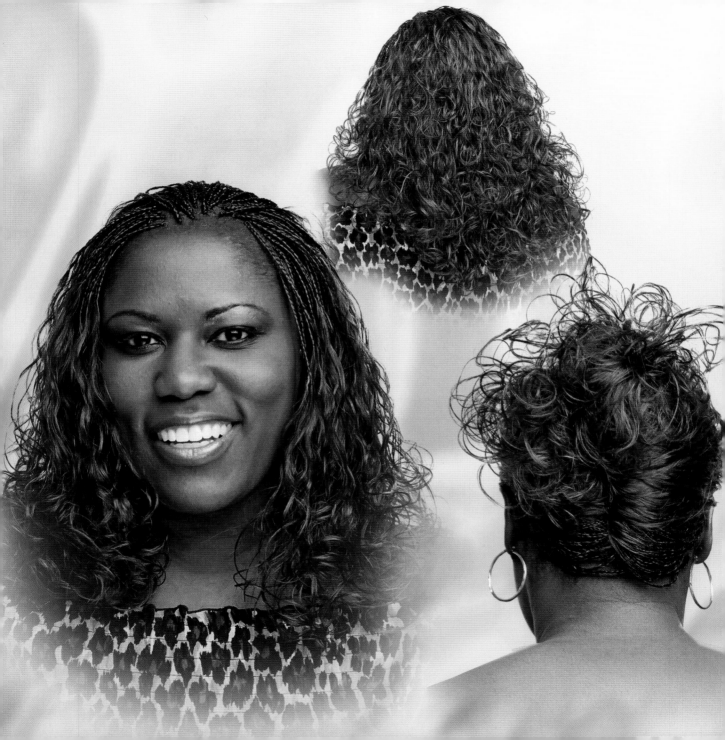

Micro Individuals

The same technique is used for micro individuals as for the individuals on the previous page, but the hair is divided into much smaller sections, to create tiny (micro) braids. The images on the left show micro individuals using two-tone deep-wave human hair. On the right are micro individuals created with long, bone-straight human hair. At top right, the braids are pulled back, and the loose ends are coiled at the top of the head, almost like a bun above a crown of braids.

Caring for Your Hair

To remove micro-braided human hair:
1. Cut the human hair past the point where the natural hair ends. This should be the same place where the nail glue was placed when the braids were put in. Be sure not to cut your own natural hair.
2. Shampoo natural hair three times.
3. Apply conditioner and leave it in to make the next few steps easier.
4. Hold between five and ten micro braids in one hand; with the other hand use a fine-tooth comb to gently comb through the braids. Begin at the end of the hair and move gradually toward the scalp as you comb out the braids.
5. Completely comb through one group of braids before moving on to the next section of braids.

INDIVIDUALS

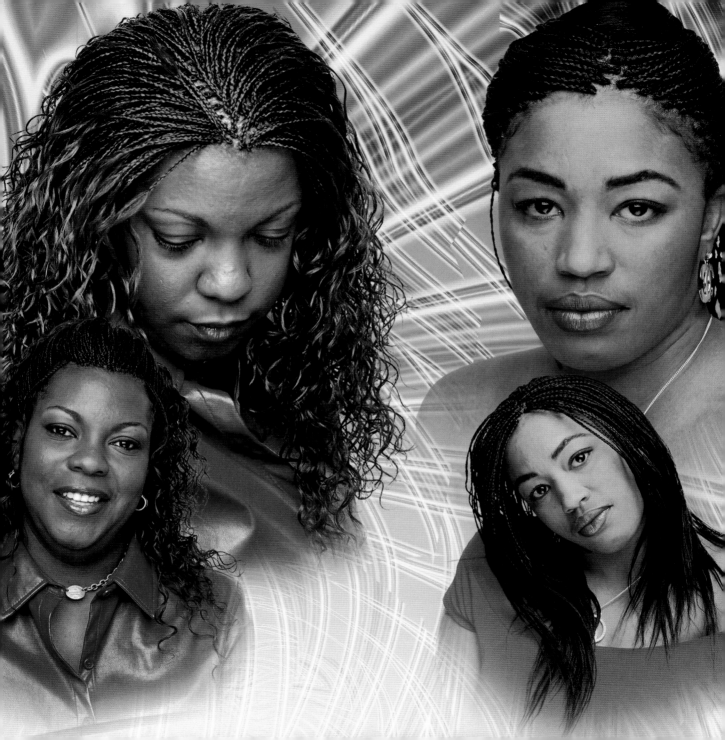

Hair lacing, because it is essentially braids, can be left in the same amount of time as individuals—about two months.

The look of hair lacing is similar to that of invisible cornrows. Human hair is attached to the natural hair with braids. The human hair, which camouflages the braids, hangs loose from the braids. See the step-by-step instructions on page 14 to learn this technique.

Bone Straight and Wet and Wavy

In the three left-hand photos, showing bone-straight yaki human hair, the hair is left to hang naturally or pulled into a French twist adorned with ornamental sticks. At right, the hair used is wet and wavy yaki human hair, left out for a full, natural look.

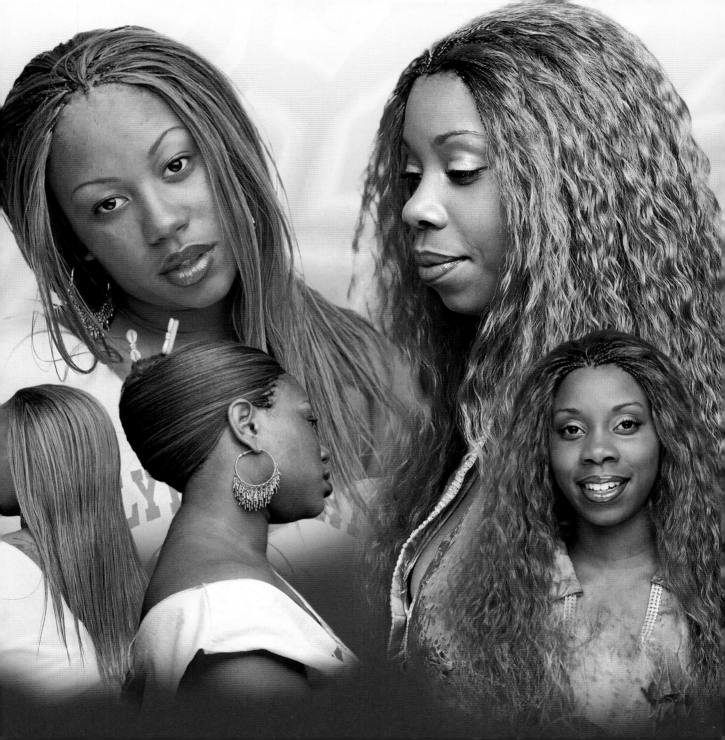

Bone Straight

In these hair-lacing shots, we get a peek at the hidden braids that hold the human hair to the natural hair, and a close-up of the French twist shown on the previous page.

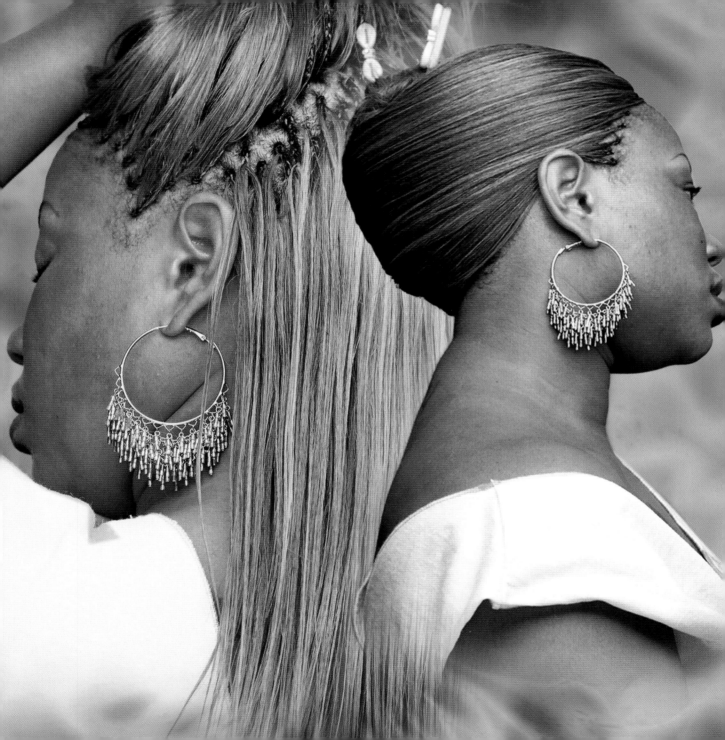

Invisible braids, like hair lacing, can be left in about two months. The wearer's natural hair must be short, though— between one and three inches long. The human or synthetic hair is simply braided tightly into the natural hair, and then allowed to hang loose once the braid has passed the ends of the natural hair.

Deep Wave

The look of invisible braids is similar to that of hair lacing (see page 86).

The hairstyle shown here, created with water wave human hair, while it is easy

to maintain, gives its wearer a strong, dramatic look.

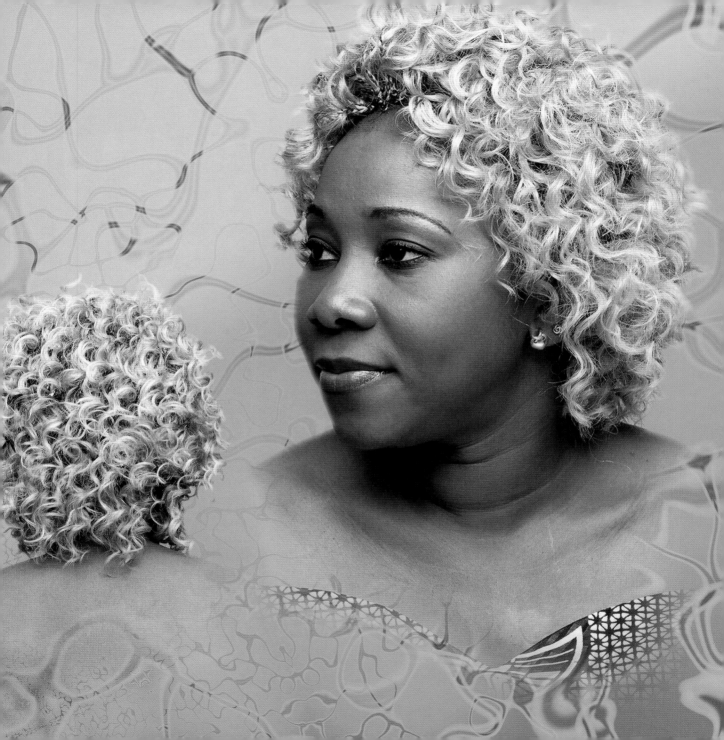

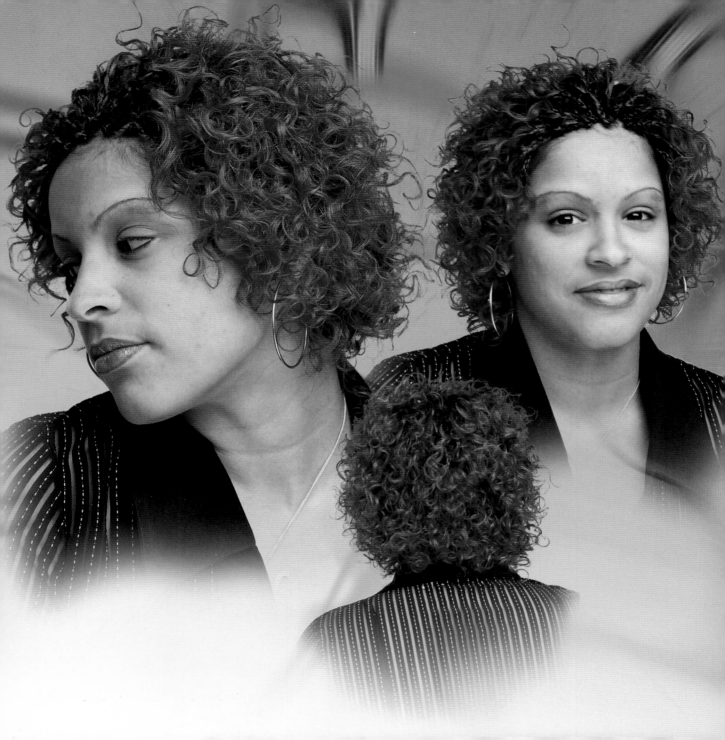

Short and Curly

This curly hair, called Diva Curl and cut off a weave track, creates a dramatic style all its own with its strong curls and bold color, but it can also be pulled back in a clip to give its wearer a little variety.

INVISIBLE BRAIDS

Wild Hair

This hairstyle, made with Afro-curl hair cut off a weave track, is for the more daring set. Its wearer portrays a strong, independent, free spirit when the style is worn loose, but it can be tamed with a barrette or two for more staid events.

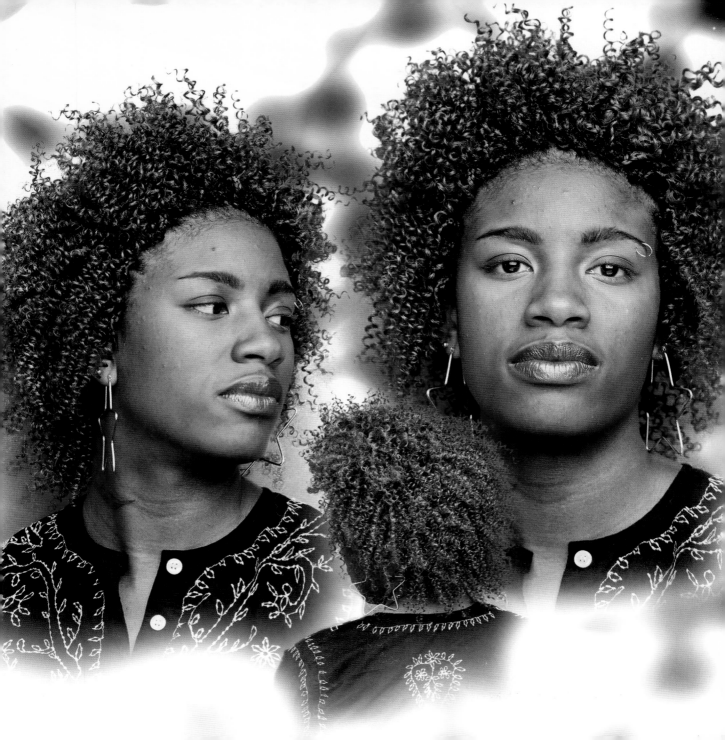

Medium-Length Natural Look

This hairstyle, created with deep wave hair, perfectly marries style with a natural, casual look. It looks comfortable and relaxed but can be pulled back for a more businesslike look, or strands can be allowed to fall around the face whenever its wearer channels her romantic side.

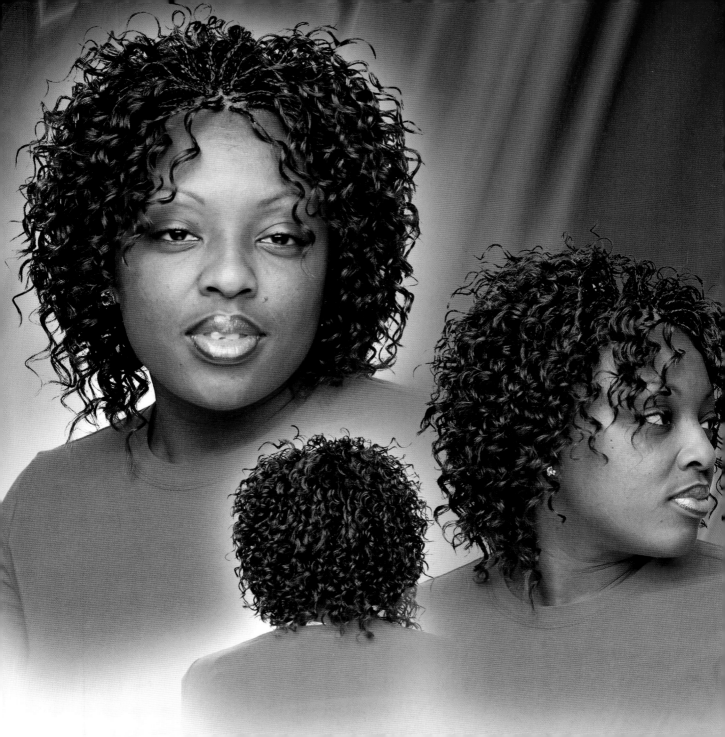

INVISIBLE BRAIDS

Spanish Wave

The hairstyle shown here, created with Spanish wave human hair, can be worn up or down, or partially up, with some locks to frame the face for a soft, romantic look.

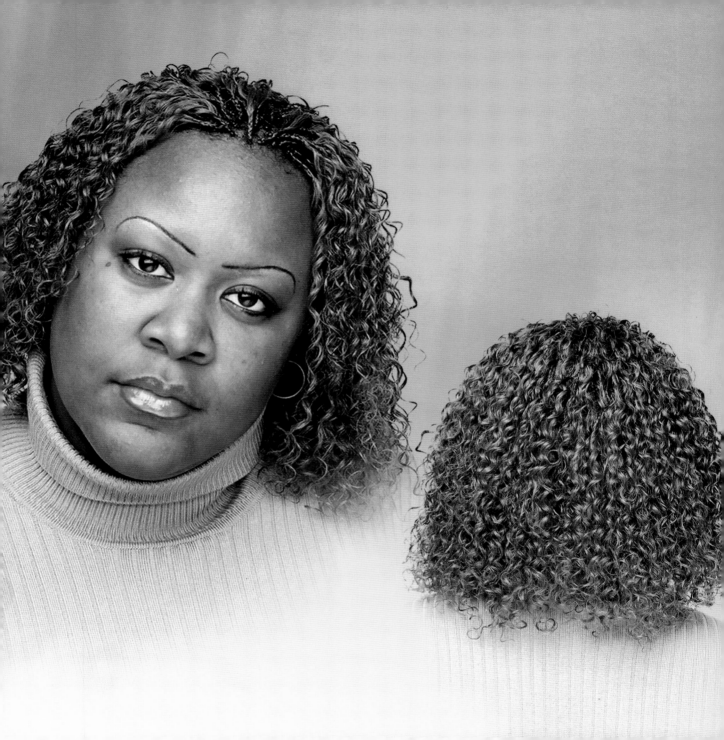

INVISIBLE BRAIDS

Curly

This hairstyle, created with paradise curl human hair, can be worn down,

as shown here, pulled back for more casual events, or up for a dressy look.

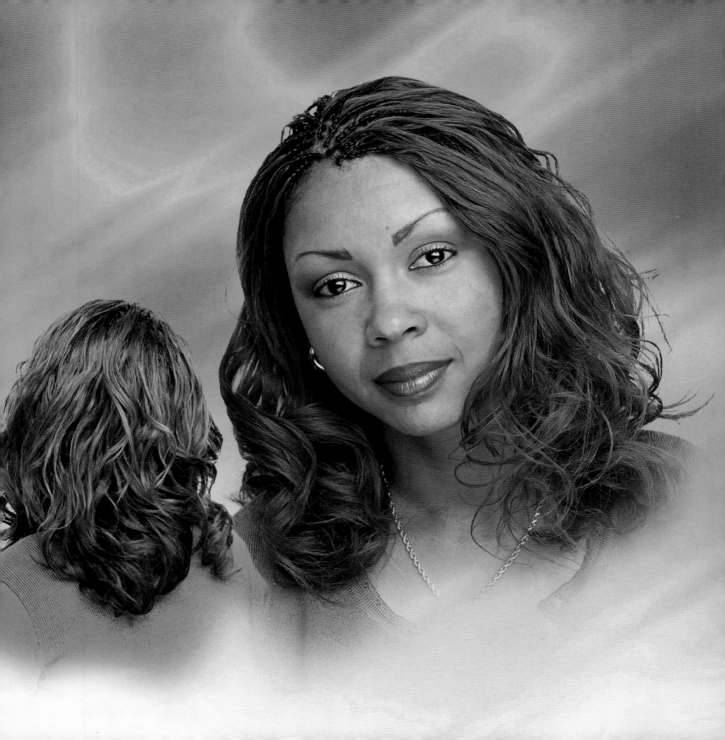

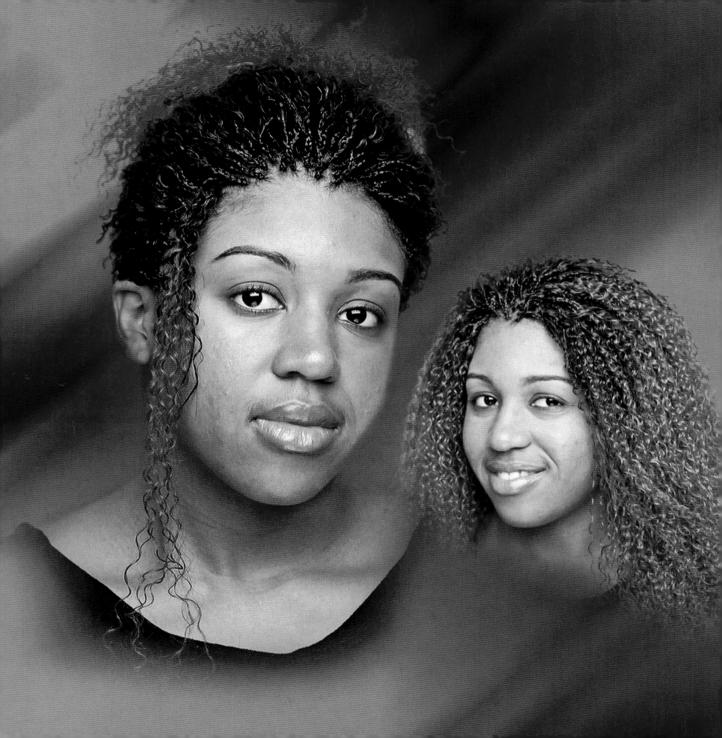

Straw Curl

This look, created with straw curl human hair, can be worn out, free and natural, as shown on the right, pulled back with some wisps around the face for a romantic look, as shown at left, or pulled up for formal occasions.

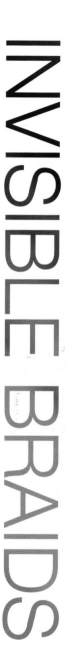

Short Wet and Wavy

Although the hair in this style is fairly short and easy to maintain, it can also be pulled back with a clip to vary the look or even with a jeweled barrette to create a dressier appearance. This style was created with spring water natural hair cut off a weave track.

tip

To wear this particular hairstyle, your natural hair must be short (between one and three inches long).

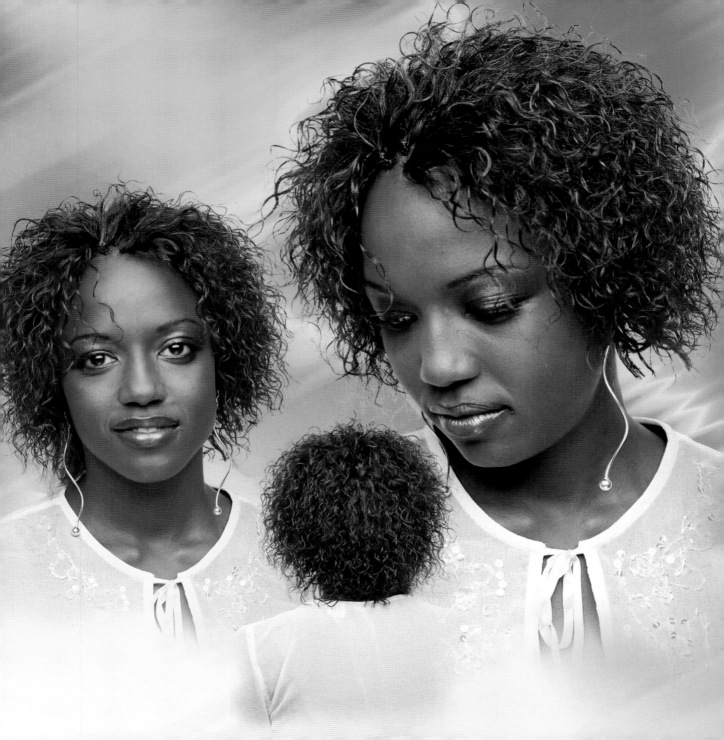

Afro Puff

This style, created with Afro puff human hair, gives a slightly wild, somewhat disheveled look. After it's washed, it looks a bit more like straw curls.

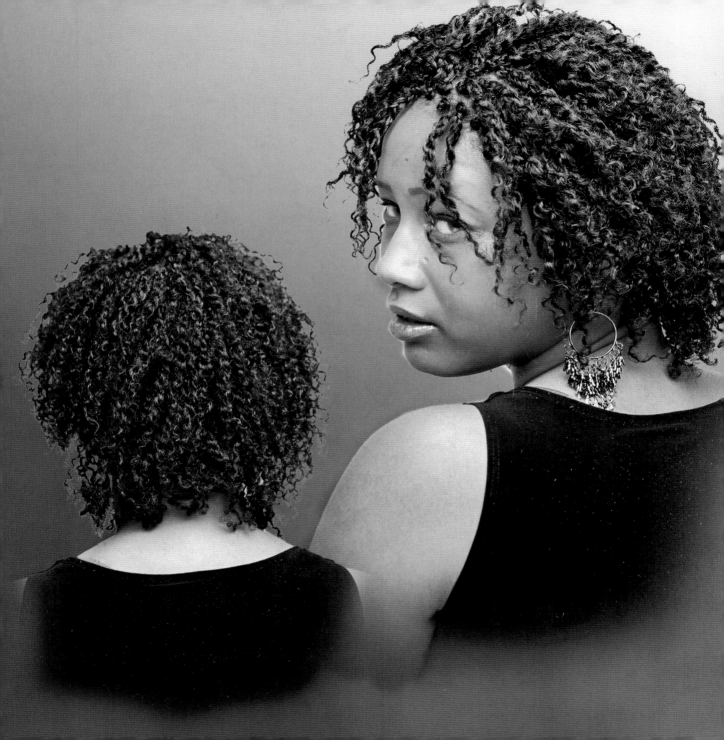

Weaves can be left in about one month. After that, the cornrows to which the weave is attached may begin to loosen, and the weave may become unstable.

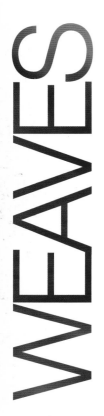

Long and Curly, Long and Straight

Weaves come in all styles and lengths. The longer styles can be pulled up and back in a myriad of ways for appropriate looks from casual to work to evening. The hair in the style on the left is called French deep curl or European curl hair. On the right is straight human hair.

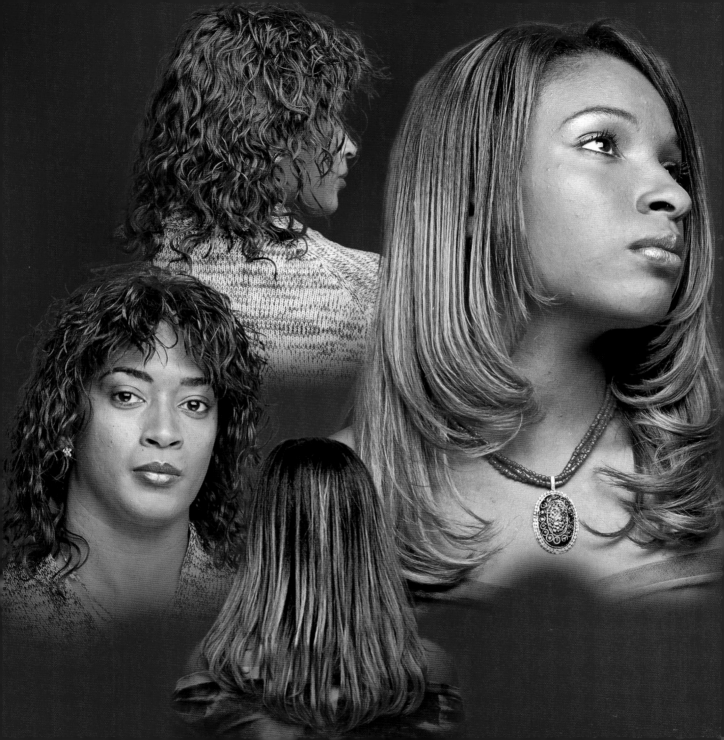

WEAVES

Short and Curly

Even the shorter weave styles, like the ones shown here, can sport a sparkly barrette or clip to dress them up for an evening out. The shoulder-length style is created with disco Jerry weave hair. The short style is created with Diva curl human hair.

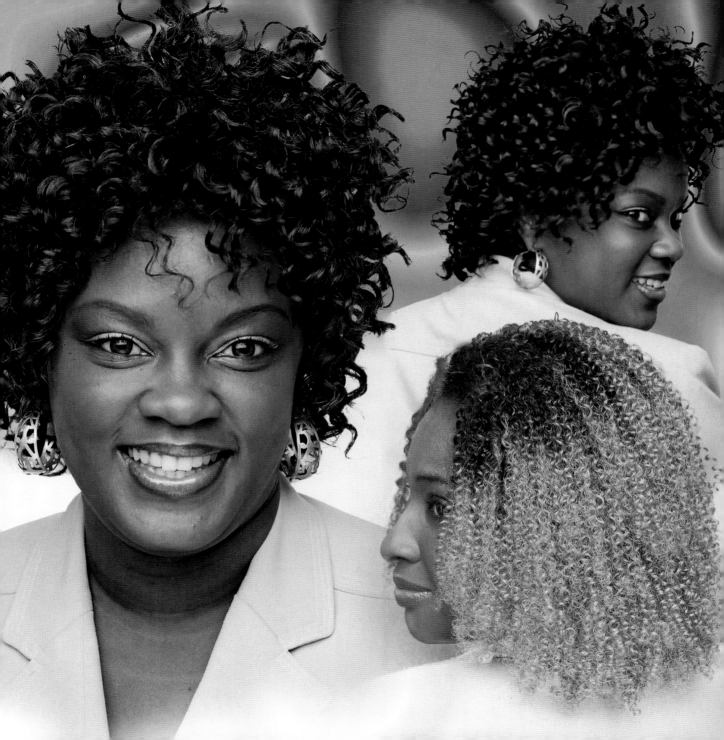

Cornrows with Weave

If you like to keep your hair short, but can't stand it hanging over your forehead or drifting across your line of sight, here's a style for you. The cornrows, which are shown angled back here but can be braided in any design you choose, keep the hair off your face, but the weave at the back gives you fullness and softness. You can even pull it back or adorn it with a clip or barrette if you desire.

tip

Hidden under the weave is a spiral of cornrows on the back of the head, onto which the weave tracks are sewn.

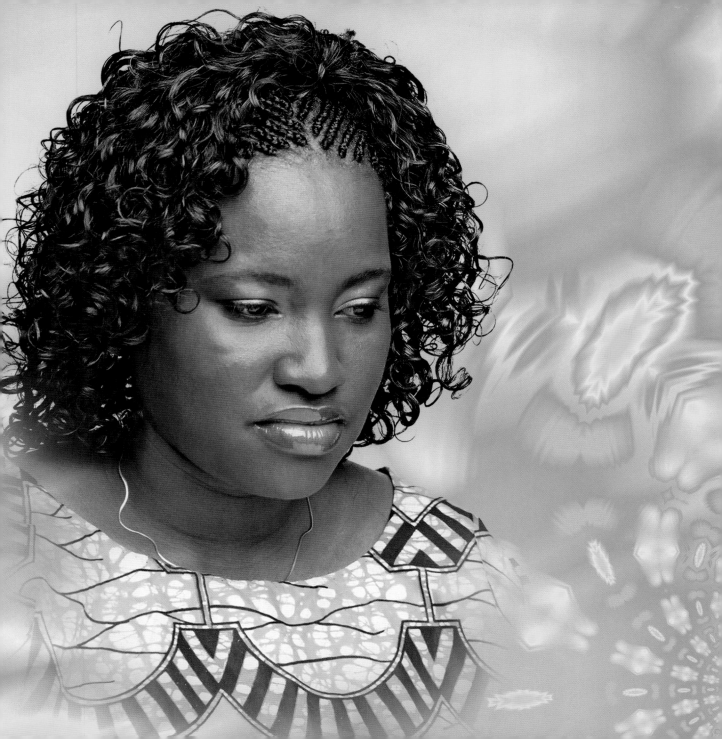

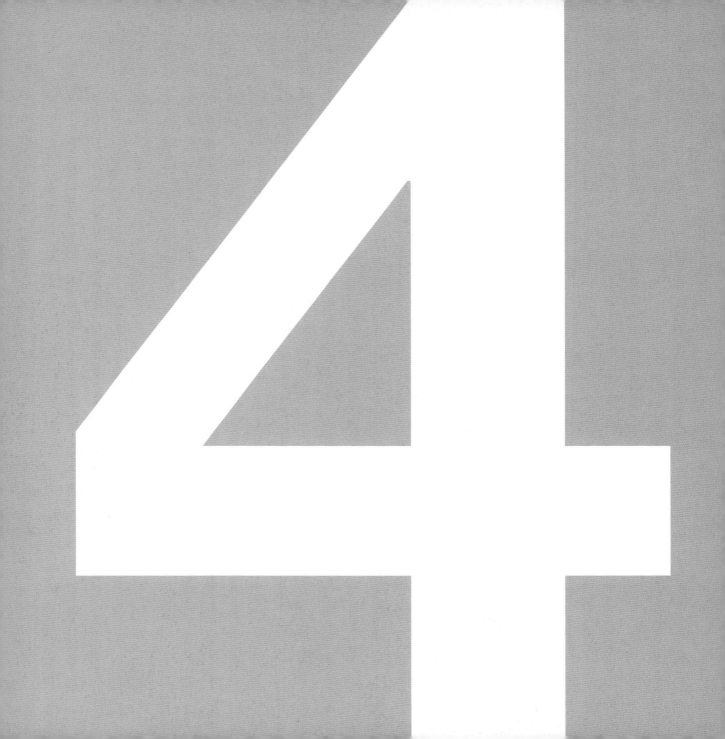

HAIRSTYLES
CREATED WITH
NATURAL HAIR

CORNROWS

Natural cornrows, just like the ones created from synthetic or human hair extensions, last about a month before they'll need to be taken out and replaced with a new style.

Zigzag Cornrows

Here is just one example of the versatility of the cornrow. In this style, groups of three cornrows are interwoven in a chainlike design, with the "chains" separated from each other by micro cornrows that travel straight from the front of the head to the back. The style finishes with the cornrows braided out to the ends.

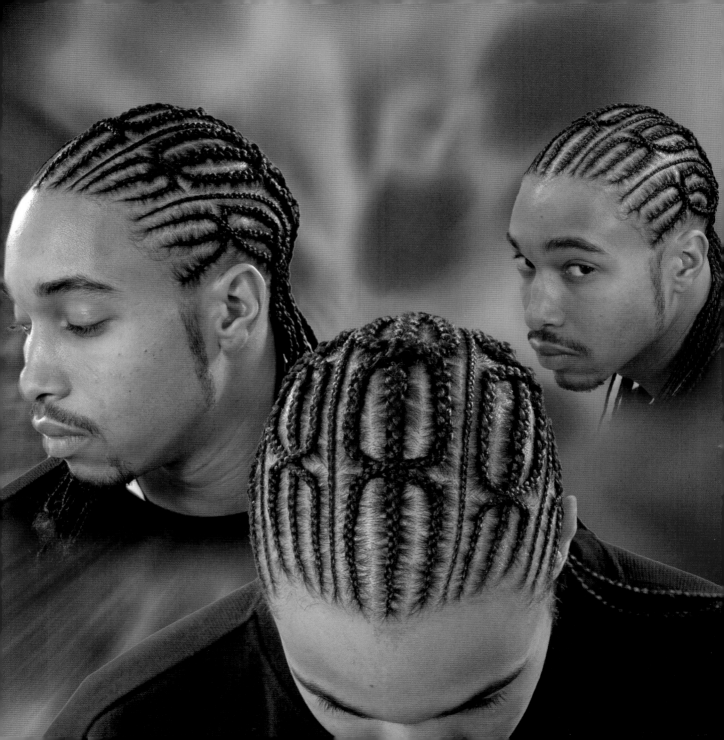

Long Cornrows

This straightforward, easy style, small cornrows that fan out from the top of the forehead to the back, keeps the wearer looking sleek and stylish.

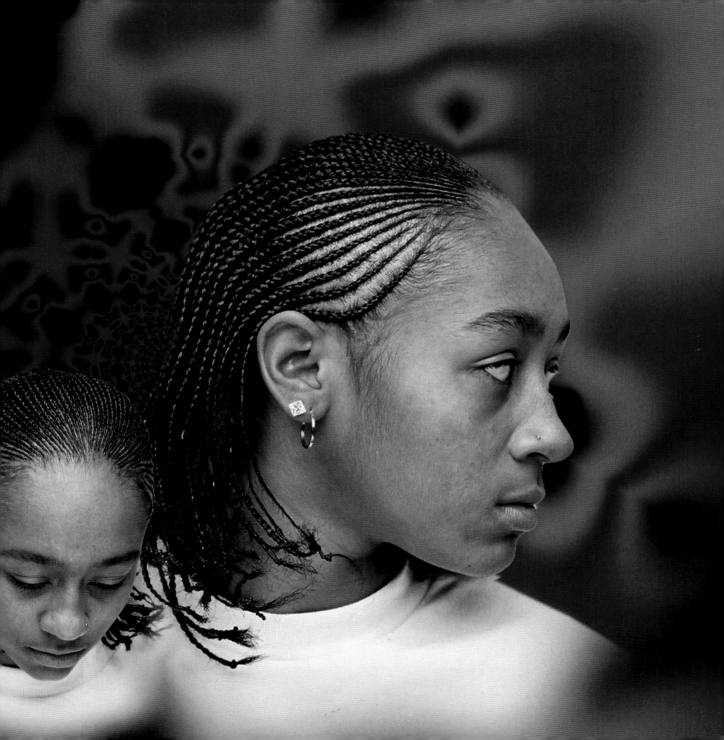

Designed Long Cornrows

This style's design is a little more complicated than the one shown on the previous page. The cornrows travel sideways instead of straight back, beginning at various points to the side of the center of the head, angling forward and then back, and ending in plaits curled at the end.

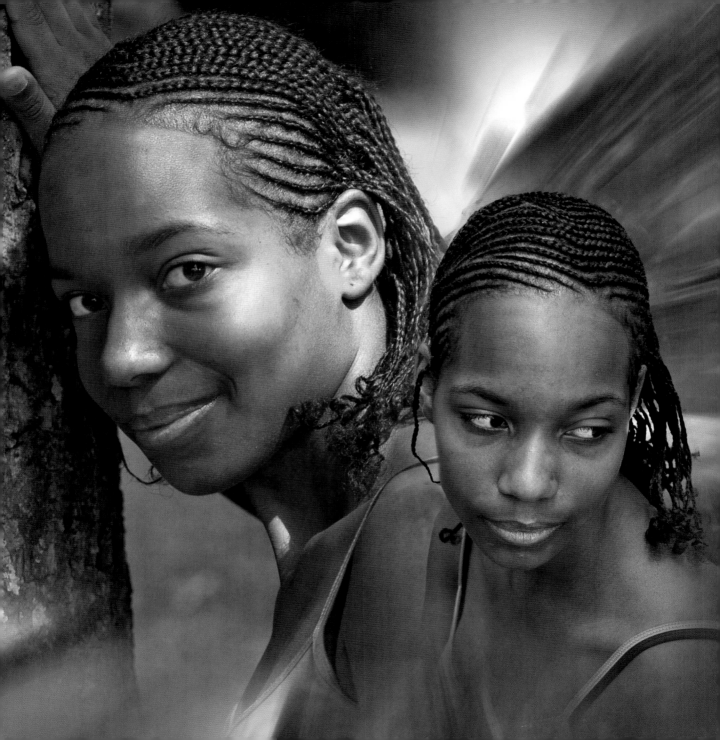

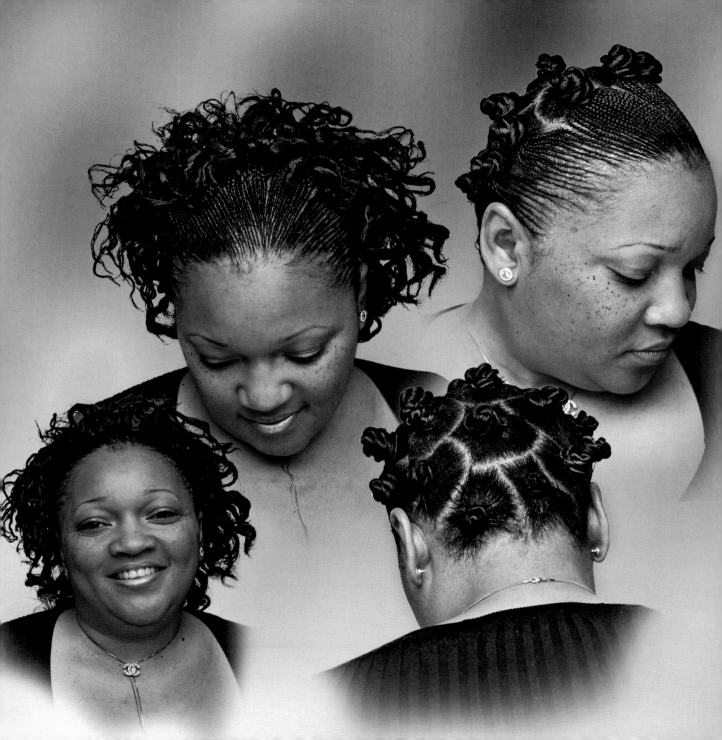

Cornrows with China Twist

The micro cornrows in this style begin traveling straight back but then angle into groups to be gathered in China twists (held with rubber bands) across the crown of the head. To complete the style, the rest of the hair is sectioned and banded into China twists as well (right-hand photos). At left, the hair at the end of the cornrows is curly and free, giving the wearer a dramatically different style choice.

CORNROWS

Natural individuals usually last about two months, like synthetic and human hair individuals. They'll have gotten a little rough by then, so you'll need to take them out and try a new style.

Short Individuals

In this natural hairstyle the hair has been carefully parted for a balanced, symmetrical result. The braids are individuals; they curl naturally at the ends.

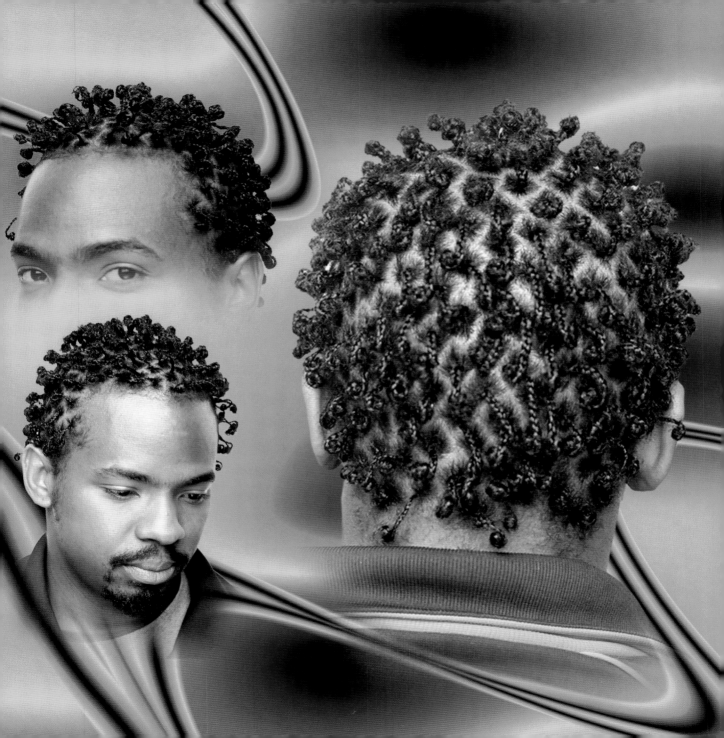

INDIVIDUALS

Long Individuals

This style is natural individuals also, but it is dramatically different from the one shown on the previous page. Here the hair is parted vertically into large sections around the head, and then the hair is divided into smaller horizontal sections for the individual braids. This hair is much longer, so the braids hang down all around the wearer's head.

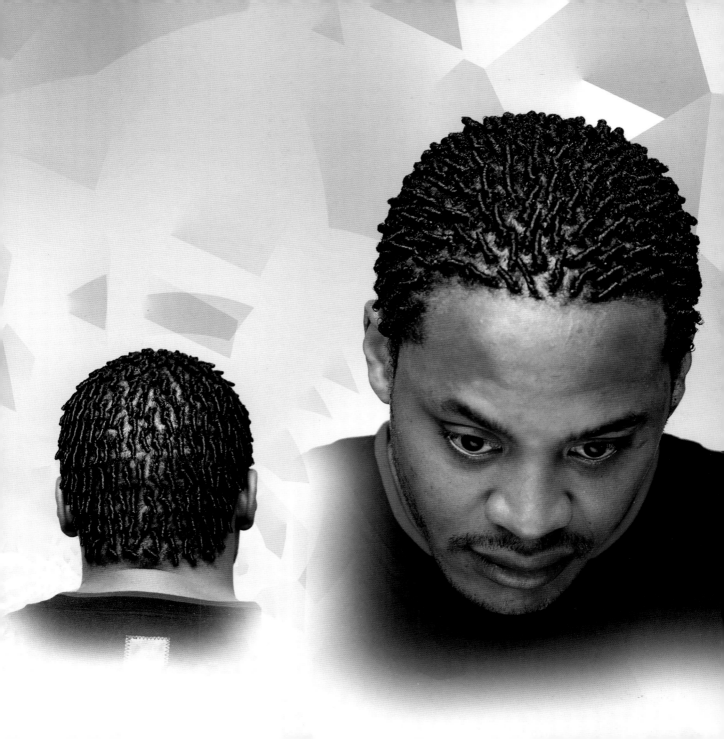

Two-Hand Twists

Two-hand twists are one of the easiest styles to create. At left and top right, the style is shown on a younger wearer, but the style works well for any age, as seen on the wearer at center and bottom right.

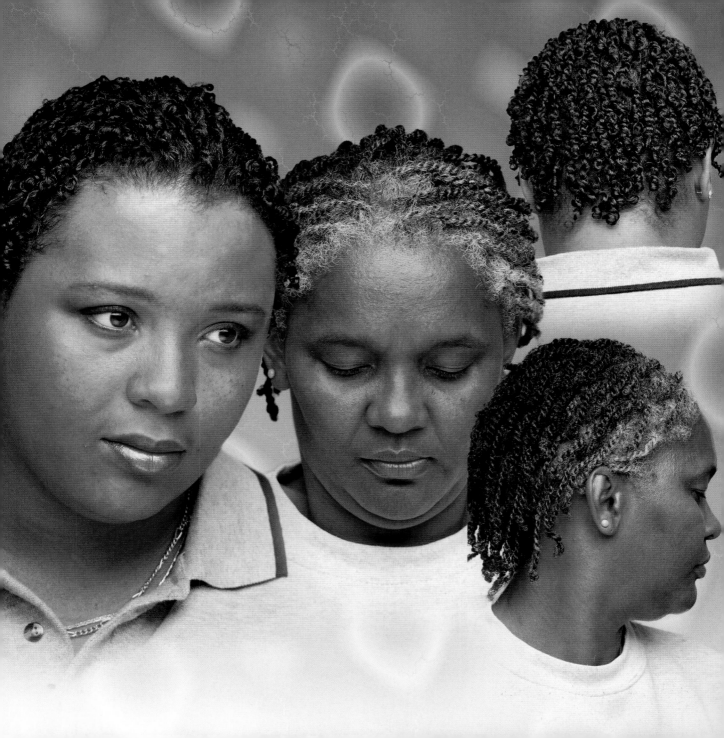

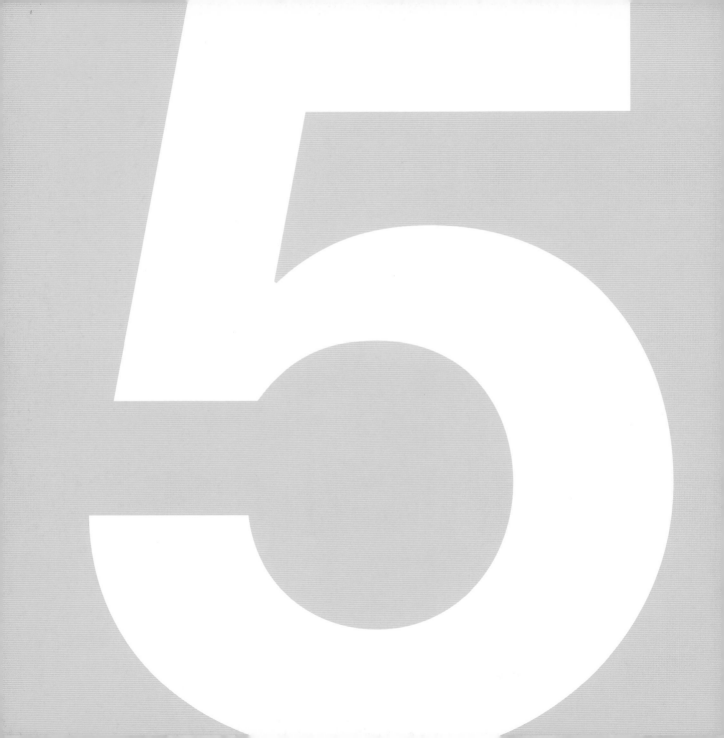

PIXIES

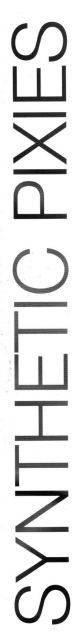

All kinds of pixies, whether they're made with synthetic hair or yarn, can be left in the same amount of time as individuals—about two months.

Long Pixies

Pixies can be twists or braids. As described in the step-by-step instructions on page 9, pixies are very tight braids or twists. They are set up like individuals and provide versatility in styling, just as individuals do. These pixies, created with synthetic hair and with the ends curled, are worn loose in the upper left- and right-hand images, but gathered back into a self-contained pony tail, with a few loose strands to frame the face, at bottom left.

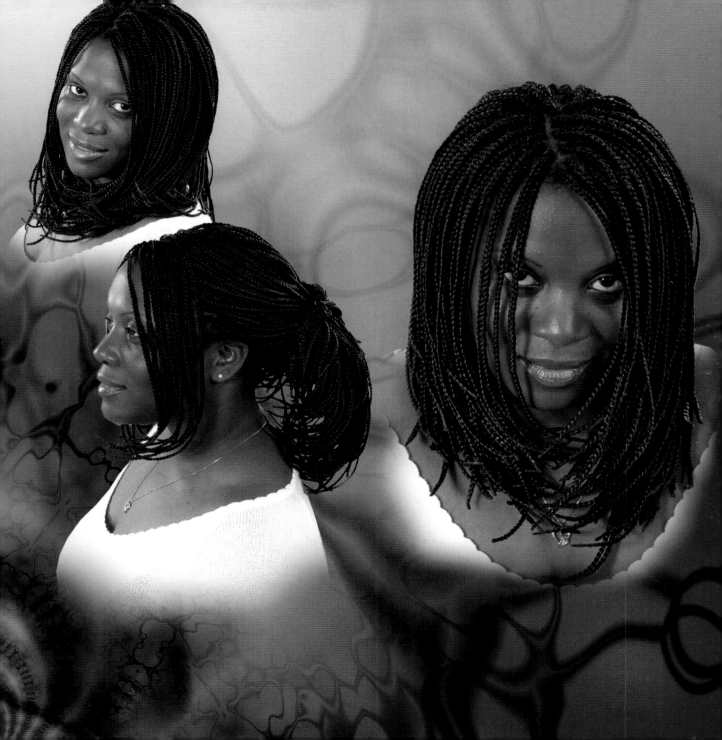

Short Senegalese Pixies

These Senegalese pixies are done with synthetic hair. They're a great style to try when you're growing your hair out or when your perm is growing old. Here they camouflage your transitioning style with a fashionable and attractive all-purpose look.

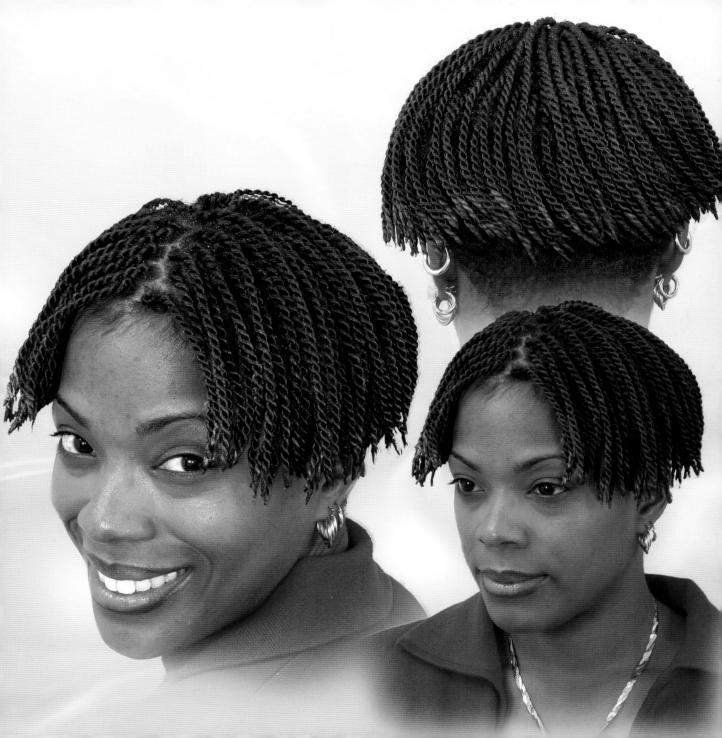

Long Senegalese Pixies

Here is an example of long Senegalese pixies, which offer the same versatility as other individual braid styles.

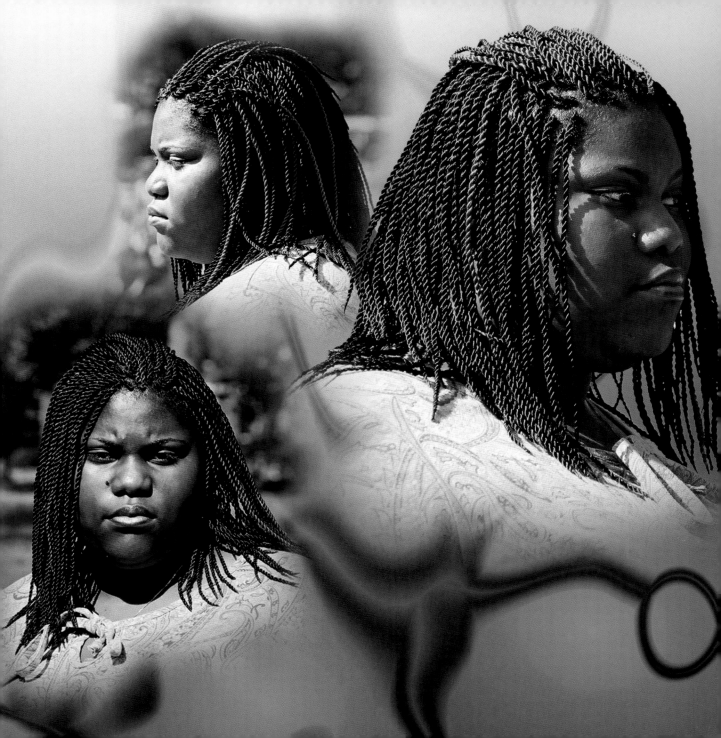

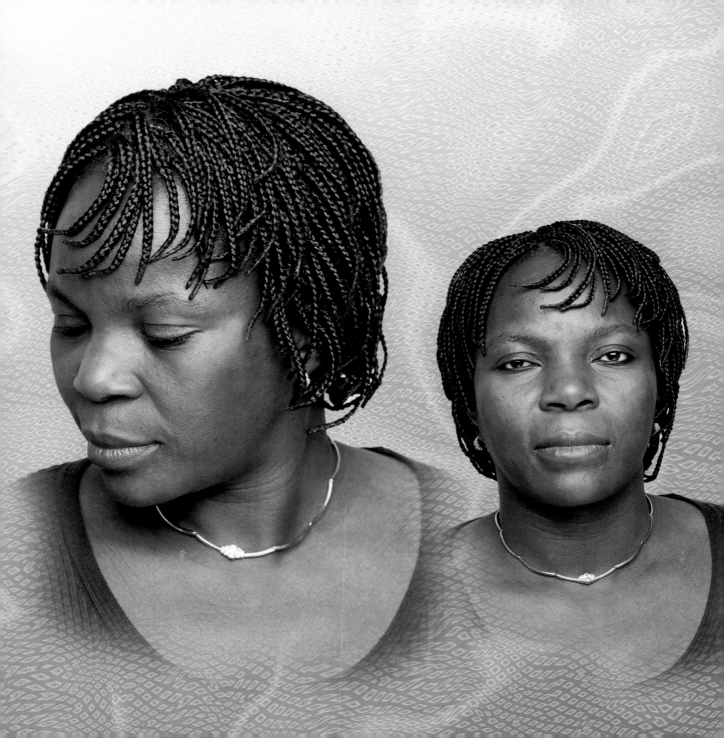

Layered Pixies

These short synthetic pixies are done in a layered style—all the added hair is the same length, but where the hair is placed on the head determines how long it looks on the wearer's head.

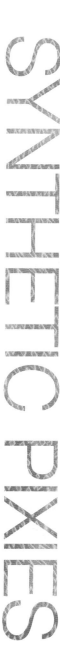

SYNTHETIC PIXIES

Pixies with Curled Ends

These pixes, made with synthetic hair, are tightly curled at the ends for a very feminine look.

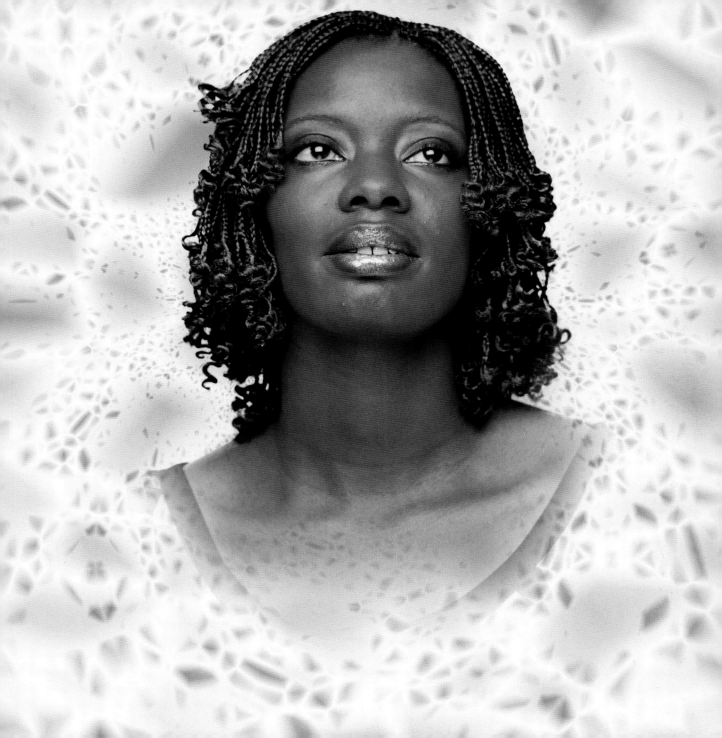

African Twist Pixies

An African twist pixie is the same as an African twist, just tighter. Synthetic two-tone hair is used here to create a style that will definitely lend an exotic element to your look.

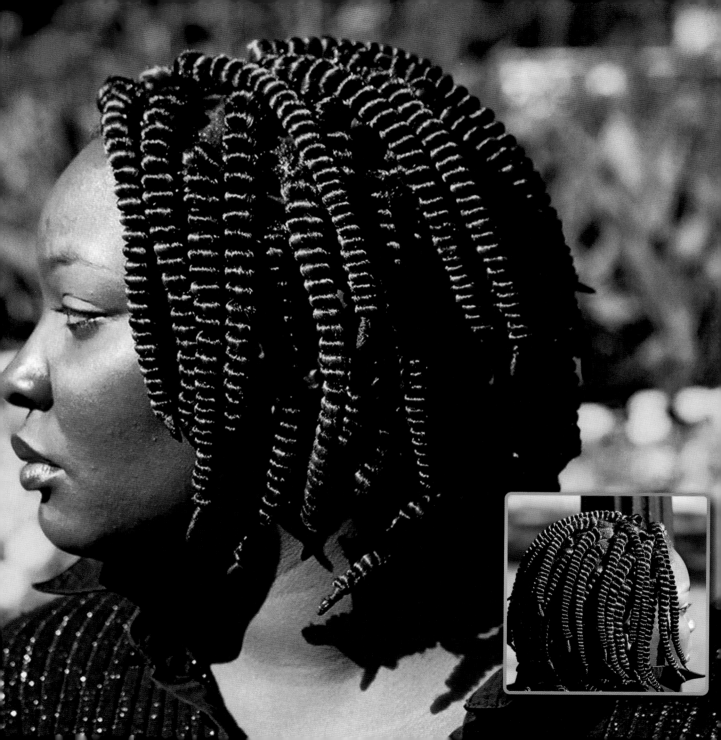

Short Yarn Pixies

Yarn pixies are done just like any other pixies, but instead of synthetic or human hair, yarn is added to the natural hair and braided or twisted in to create the hairstyle. Because the yarn will come loose if left to hang free at the end of the twist, it must be sealed with a hot curling iron at the ends to hold the pixie style.

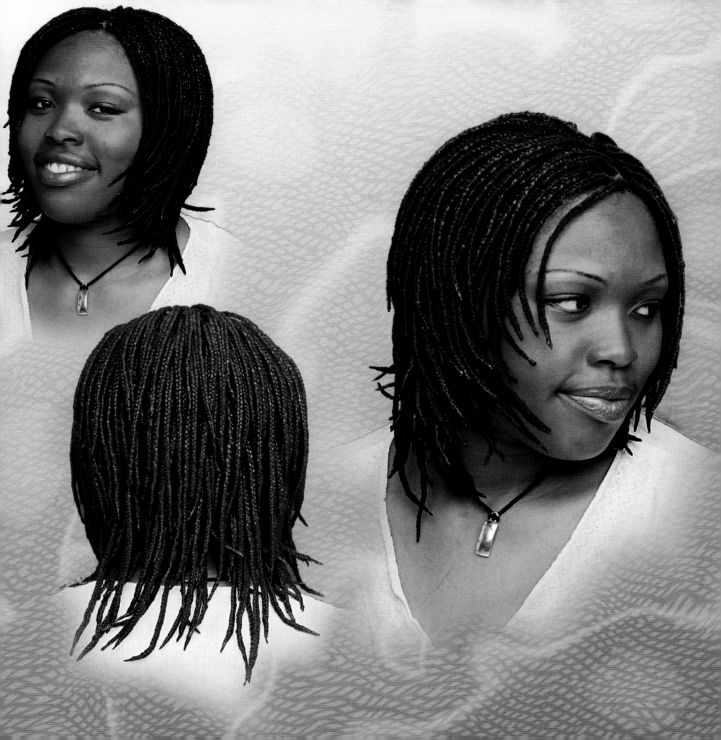

Yarn Twist Pixies

All the styles in which synthetic or human hair is added to natural hair can be long or short, as can all the styles created with yarn instead of hair, and yarn is actually easier to work with than synthetic hair. Here are examples of long and short yarn twist pixies; the ends of both show the color change created by the sealing process.

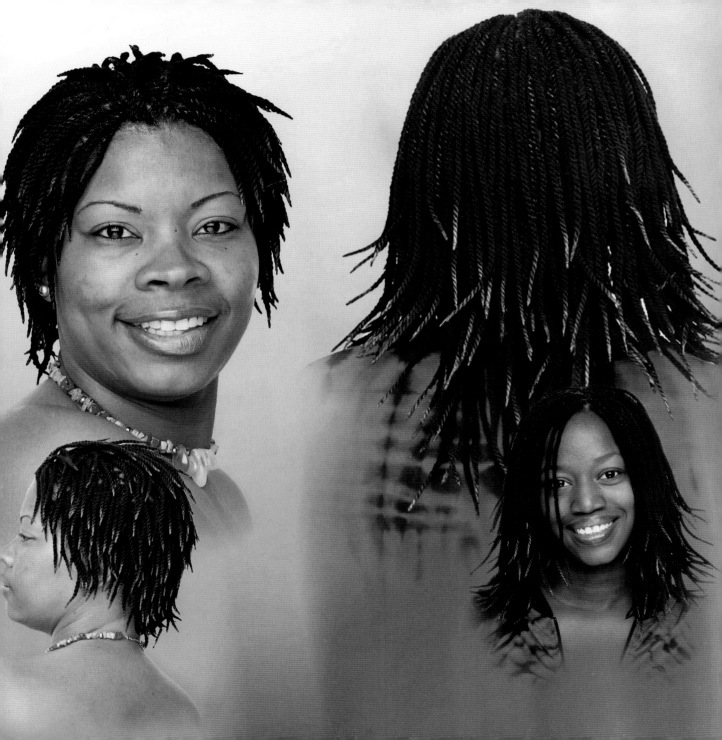

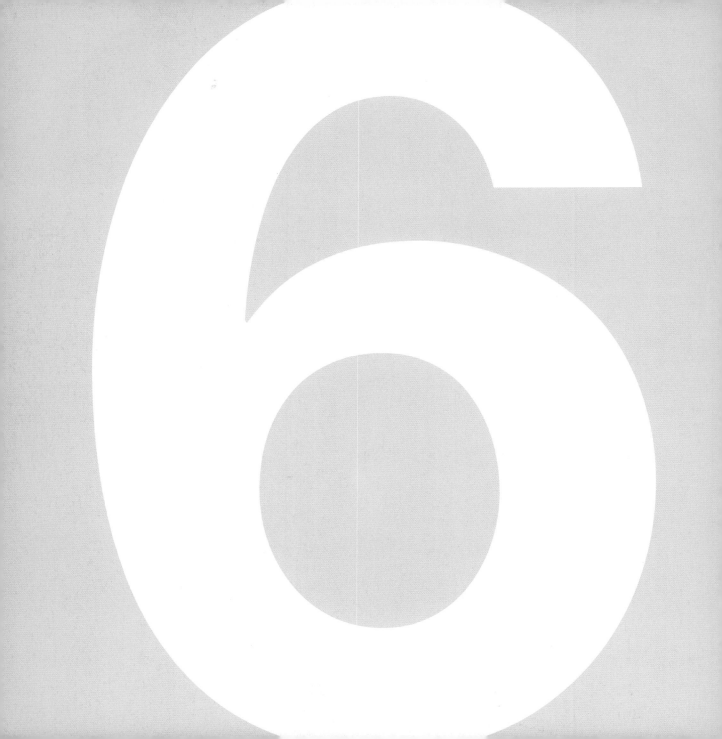

SPECIALTY HAIRSTYLES

Faa-Ling-Ying

Though it's hard to believe when you're looking at this dramatic hairstyle, it's created the same way dreadlocks are, but the hair is wrapped with thread rather than hair. The images on this page are all of the same woman; on the left the hair is coiled into a more sedate style, and on the right the hair is extended out in all directions from her head. The hair is wrapped so tightly that it almost appears to be defying gravity.

About the Style

Different regions and peoples in West Africa assign different names to this particular style. In Guinea, it's known as the faa-ling-ying style. In Togo, it's called the "tree hairstyle." Among the Loma tribe of Liberia, this style is given the expressive name *wulibah*, or the "look at me" hairstyle.

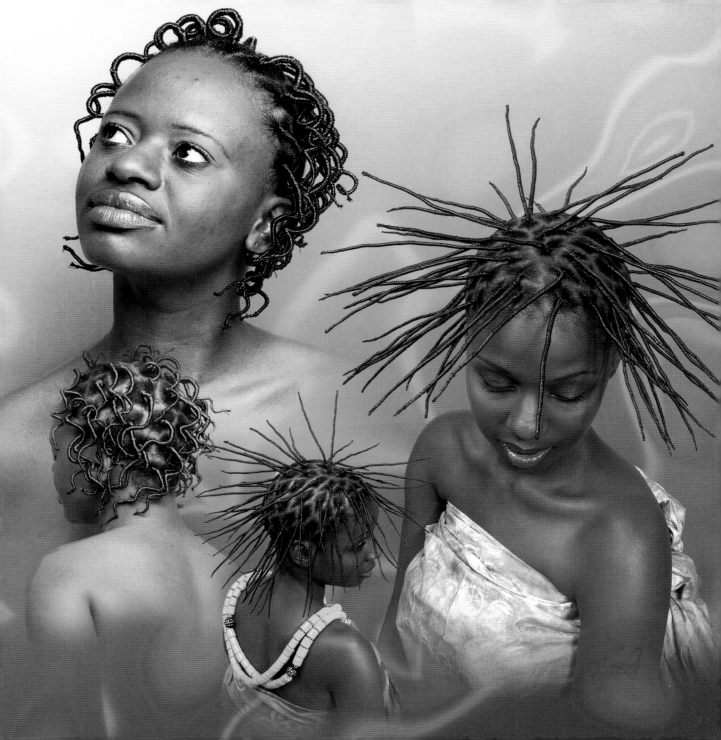

All-Natural Yolele

The yolele was a popular wedding hairstyle for Foula brides of the royal family of the Fulani tribe of West Africa. This style was also worn at special feasts and celebrations. The yolele style is made with some hair in cornrows and some hair left out, but it's done entirely with natural hair; no extensions have been added.

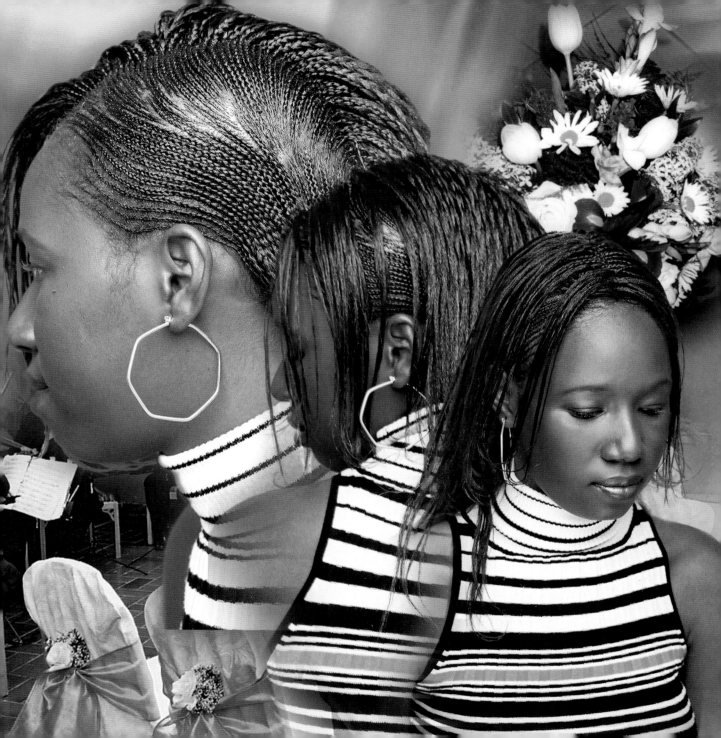

Dreadlock extensions can be left in, essentially, for the life of the wearer. Silky dreads and the faa-ling-ying style can last about two months before they begin to lose their smoothness.

Dreadlock Extensions

Refer to page 15 for step-by-step instructions on how to create dreadlock extensions. You'll need kinky human hair to create this look, which can be styled in various ways to create very different looks, as shown here.

DREADLOCKS

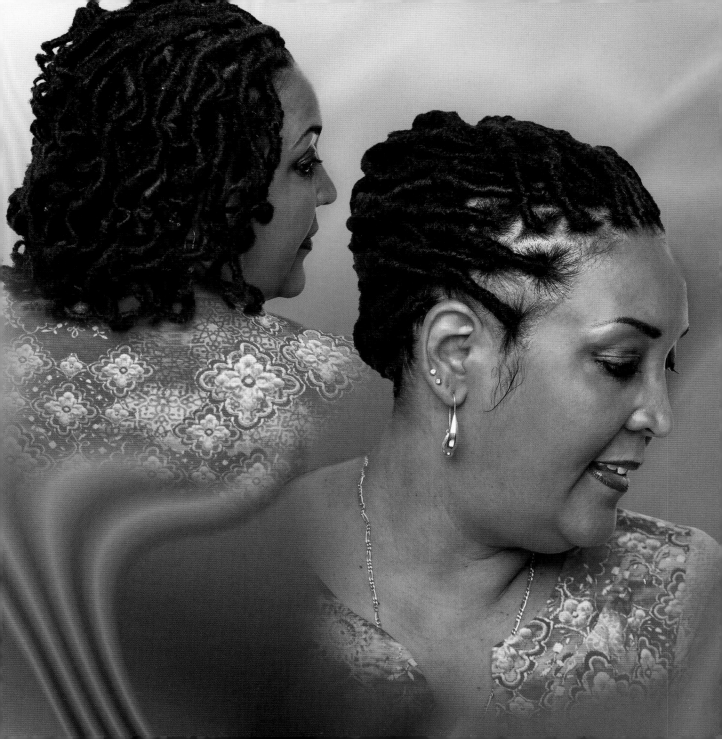

DREADLOCKS

Silky Dreads

Silky dreadlocks are created just like dreadlock extensions, but synthetic hair rather than kinky human hair is used to wrap the natural hair. The hair is wrapped tightly here, too, as in the faa-ling-ying style, as the dreads can be left straight or coiled. Here they are adorned with beads as well.

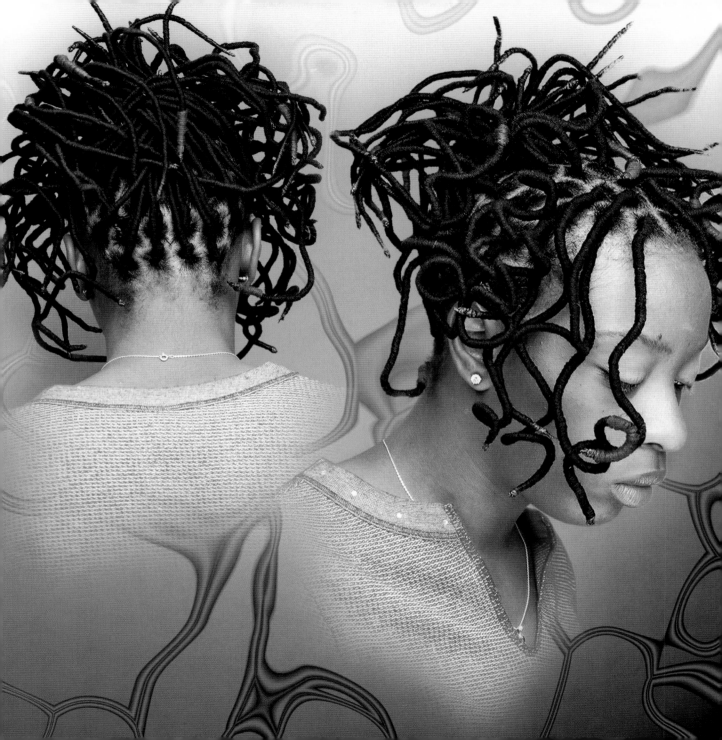

The goddess braid usually lasts only about one to two weeks. These large braids tend to get fuzzy rather quickly. The goddess braid weave, however, can last up to two months.

Goddess Braids and Fishtail Goddess Braid Weaves

At left, the goddess braids are created as described in the step-by-step instructions on page 17. In the two right-hand photos, the fishtail goddess braid weave, the goddess braids are prepackaged. The natural hair is styled in cornrows in the design you've planned for the goddess braids. You have simply to create the design with cornrows and sew the prebraided goddess braids to the cornrows.

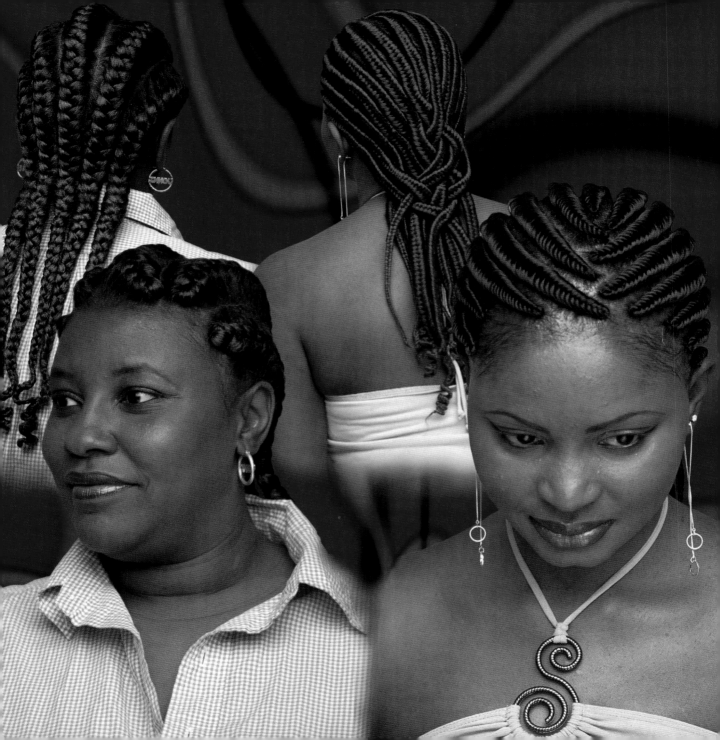

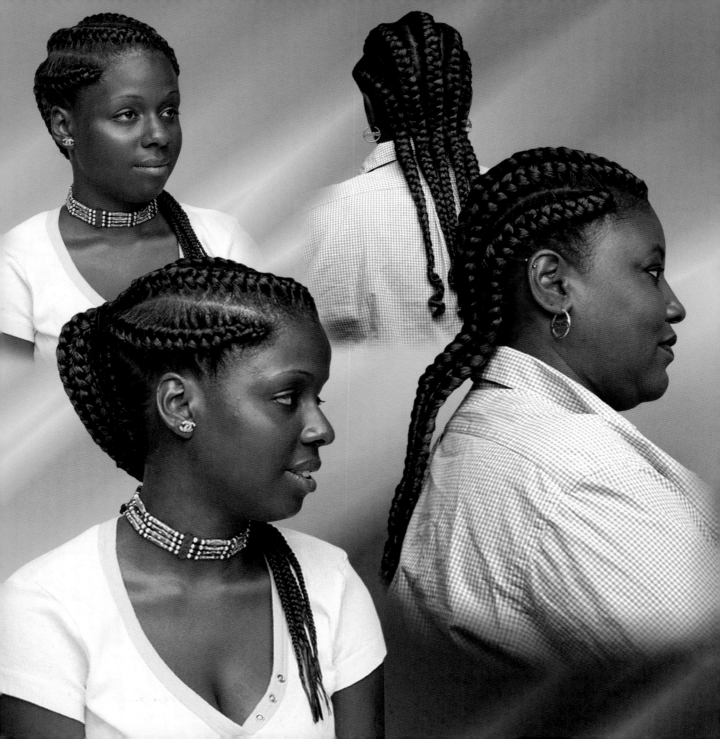

Goddess Braids

Here again are two versions of goddess braids. At left, the braids are slightly curved along the top of the head. The braids begun at the top stop at the back of the head, and additional braids are started at the neckline and braided up toward the top of the head to finish the look. At right, the goddess braids continue straight from the front hairline to the neckline and are then braided out and curled at the ends.

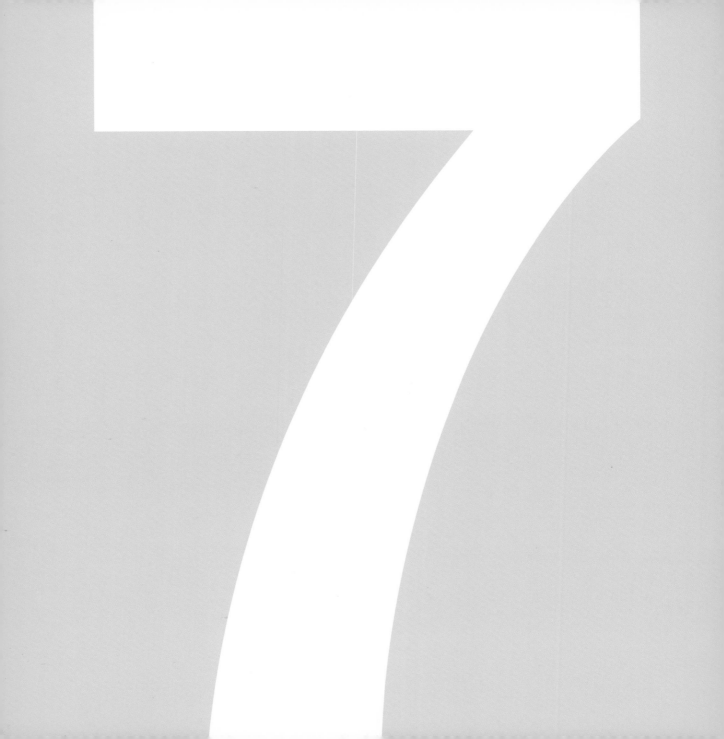

CHILDREN'S HAIRSTYLES

Just like grownups, kids can leave their cornrows in for about a month before they start to look a little worn out. Because they're kids, though, and kids can be rough on their hair, they may need refreshing even earlier.

Zigzag Cornrows

This little girl is wearing cornrows that begin all along the hairline and along the zigzag part and always end at the point the ponytail is created. Here the braids, made from pony hair, are gathered into ponytails, then knotted to hold them in place. The ends are left long and loose.

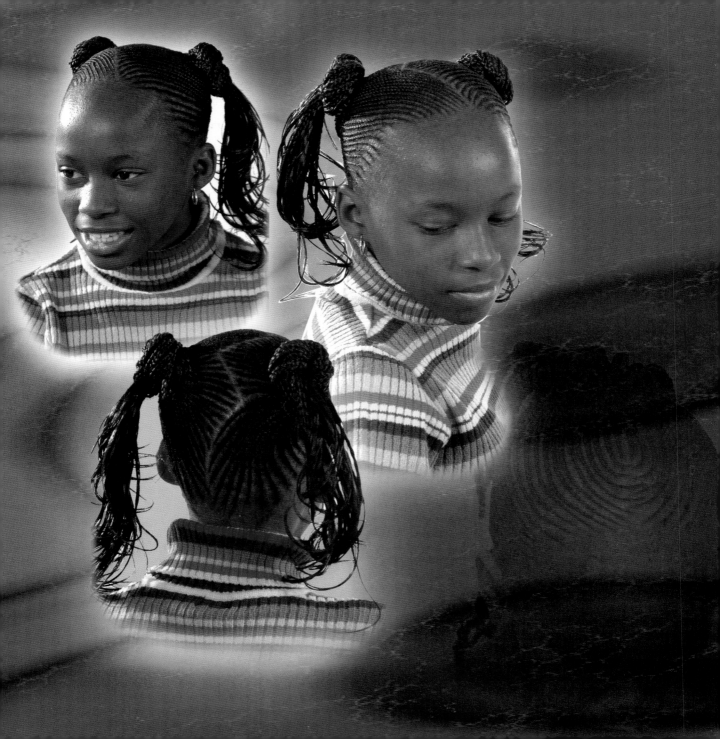

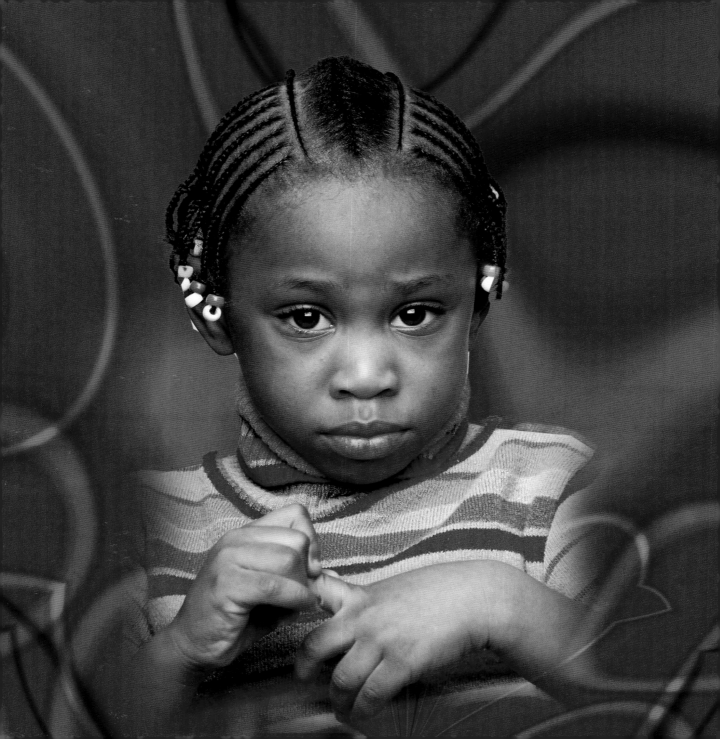

Natural Cornrows with Fishtail Goddess Braid

The centerpiece of this style is the fishtail goddess braid at the center top of the head. It's bordered by two micro cornrows. To finish, little cornrows are braided down the sides, their ends decorated with beads.

CORNROWS

Cornrows and Kinky Twists

In this multifaceted style using synthetic hair, cornrows are created at the front.

They finish as kinky twists, which are curled at the ends for a frilly, girly look.

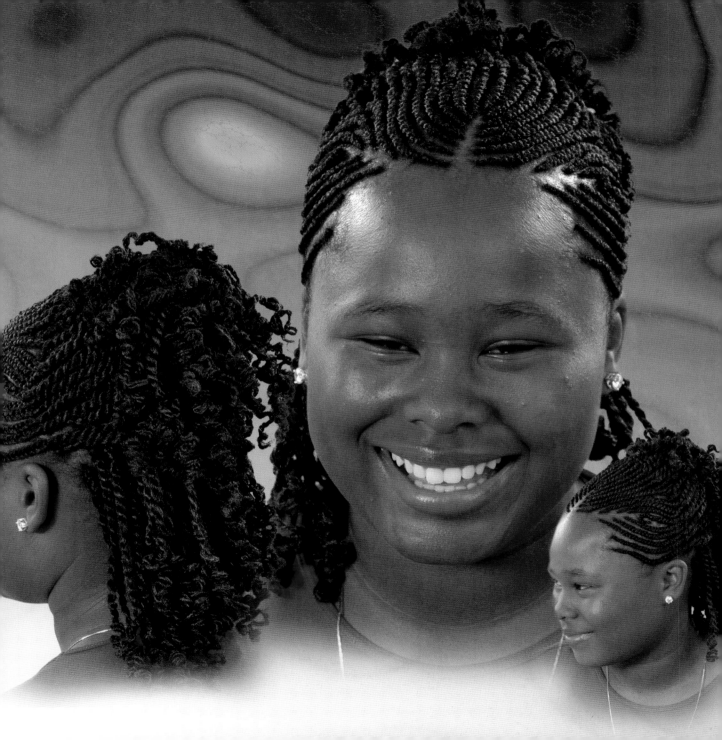

CORNROWS

Cornrows with Senegalese Twists

These geometrically designed cornrows, created with synthetic hair, end as Senegalese twists, curled at the end. This style, just like the other children's styles, is good for everyday wear, including sports, but can be dressed up with curls or tied up or back with a pretty ornament to dress it up.

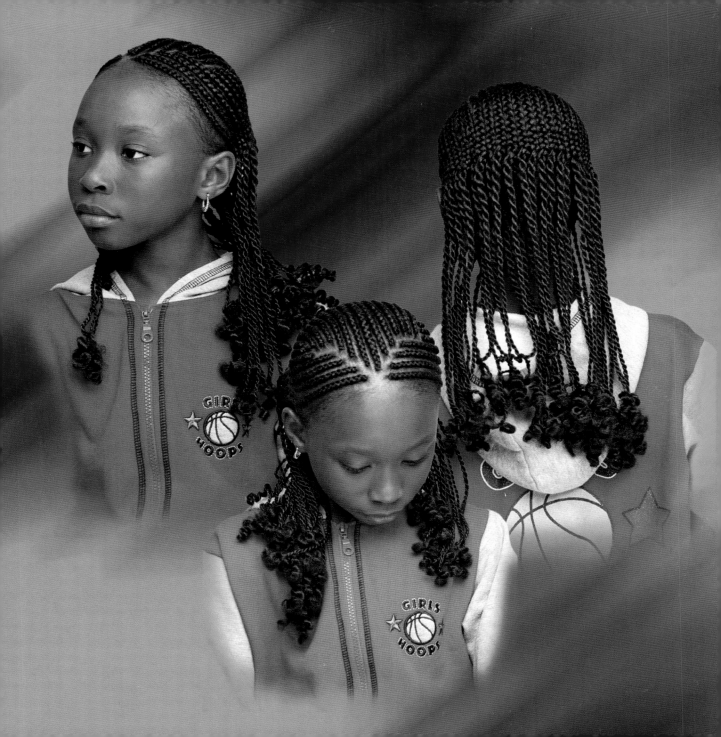

Twists can be left in for about two months before they start to show their age. For children, though, who can be a little harder on their hair than adults are, the style may need freshening up before two months go by.

TWISTS

Nubian Twists

These Nubian twists are created with synthetic hair and left loose for an adorable natural look.

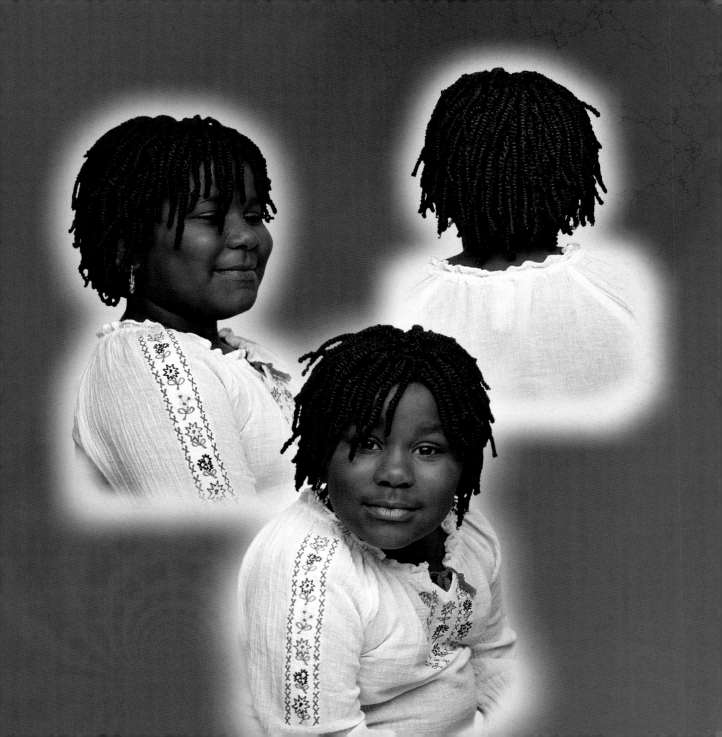

Afro Puff Twists

These Afro puff twists, created with synthetic hair, can be worn down,

as shown here, or clipped back for special events.

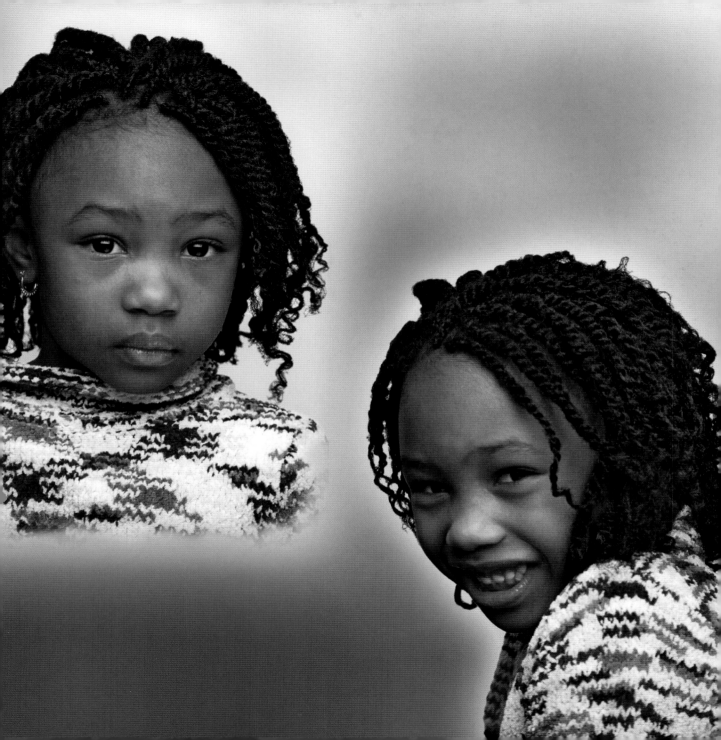

Individuals for kids usually last about two months, just as they do for adults, but sometimes kids can be a little rougher on their hair than adults are, so the style may need some attention a little earlier.

Long, Large Individuals

Extra character is added to these large individuals by the inclusion of randomly spaced beads and corkscrew curls at the ends.

INDIVIDUALS

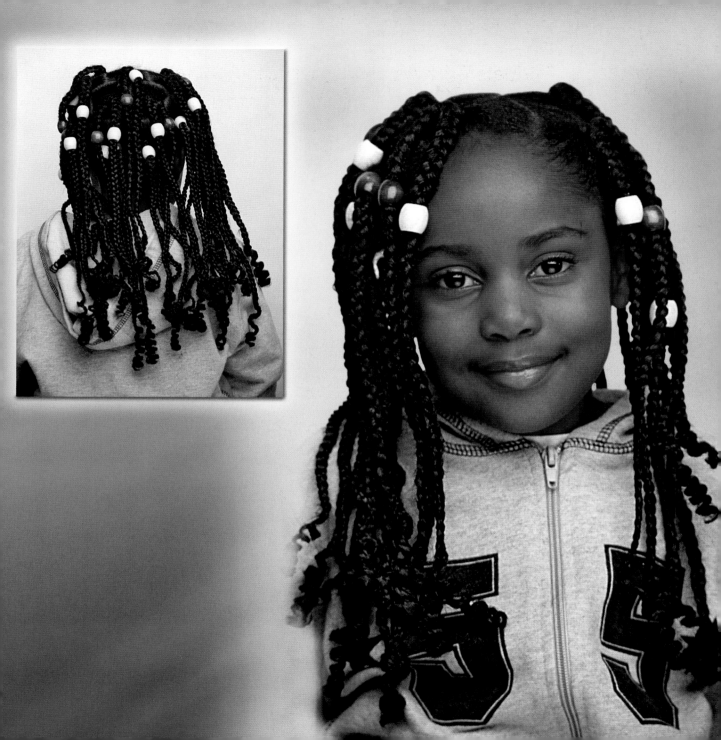

Sisters in Braids

The little girl on the left is wearing individuals pulled into two ponytails and curled on the ends for an adorable go-to-school style. Her little sister, in the middle, is wearing natural micro cornrows with a Nubian twist in the back (visible over her right shoulder). On the right, the oldest sister is wearing designed cornrows, angled from back to front. All these styles are "shake-and-go," so the kids won't have to rush in the morning or stay up late at night to get their hair done.

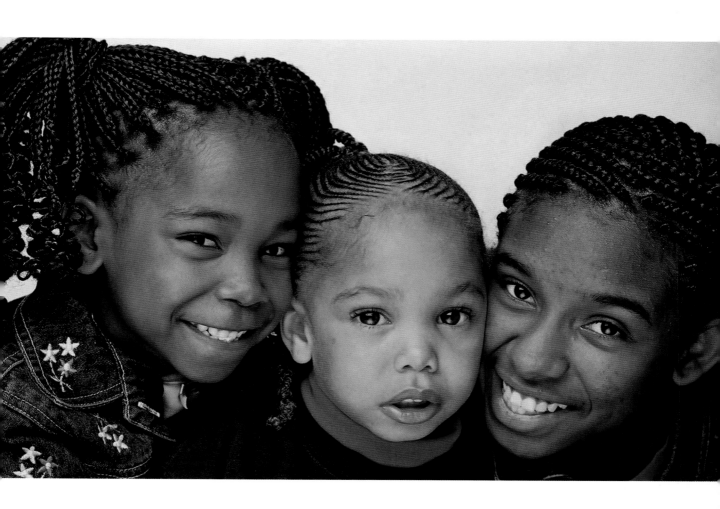

INDEX